DEATH ON HEMODIALYSIS: PREVENTABLE OR INEVITABLE?

DEVELOPMENTS IN NEPHROLOGY

Volume 35

Death on Hemodialysis:
Preventable or Inevitable?

Edited by

ELI A. FRIEDMAN
State University of New York,
Health Science Center at Brooklyn,
New York, USA

Sponsored by

The International Society for Artificial Organs

SPRINGER-SCIENCE+BUSINESS MEDIA, B.V.

Library of Congress Cataloging-in-Publication Data

```
Death on hemodialysis : preventable or inevitable? / edited by E.A.
  Friedman.
       p.    cm. -- (Developments in nephrology ; v. 35)
    ISBN 978-0-7923-2652-6      ISBN 978-94-011-0806-5 (eBook)
    DOI 10.1007/978-94-011-0806-5
    1. Hemodialysis--Congresses.  2. Chronic renal failure--Mortality-
  -Congresses.   I. Friedman, Eli A., 1933-   . II. Series.
    [DNLM: 1. Hemodialysis--mortality--congresses.  2. Risk Factors-
  -congresses.   W1 DE998EB v. 35 1994 / WJ 378 D285 1994]
  RC901.7.H45D43  1994
  617.4'61059--dc20
  DNLM/DLC
  for Library of Congress                                93-42588
```

ISBN 978-0-7923-2652-6

Printed on acid-free paper

Table of Contents

List of main authors

M. M. Avram, MD, FACP
Clinical Professor of Medicine
SUNY Health Science Center at Brooklyn
Chief, Division of Nephrology
The Long Island College Hospital
Brooklyn, NY, USA

Robert H. Barth, MD
Assistant Professor of Medicine
SUNY Health Science Center at Brooklyn
Chief, Hemodialysis,
Brooklyn V.A. Medical Center
Brooklyn, NY, USA

Geoffrey M. Berlyne, MD
Professor of Medicine
SUNY Health Science Center at Brooklyn
Chief, Nephrology Division
Brooklyn V.A. Medical Center
Brooklyn, NY, USA

Christopher R. Blagg, MD
Professor of Medicine
Division of Nephrology
University of Washington
Executive Director
Northwest Kidney Centers
Seattle, Washington, USA

Edmund Bourke, MD
Professor of Medicine
Vice-Chairman, Dept. of Medicine
SUNY Health Science Center at Brooklyn
Chief, Medical Service
Brooklyn V.A. Medical Center, USA

John D. Bower, MD
Professor of Medicine,
Division of Nephrology
University of Mississippi Medical Center
Jackson, Mississippi, USA

Allan J. Collins, MD, FACP
Executive Director
Regional Kidney Disease Program
Minneapolis, Minnesota, USA

Barbara G. Delano, MD
Professor of Medicine
Director of Home Hemodialysis
SUNY Health Science Center at Brooklyn
Brooklyn, NY, USA

Eli A. Friedman, MD
Distinguished Teaching Professor
Chief, Renal Disease Division
SUNY Health Science Center at Brooklyn
Brooklyn, NY, USA

Hans J. Gurland, MD
Professor of Medicine
University of Munich
Munich, Germany

Philip J. Held, PhD
Program Director, Urban Institute
Washington, DC, USA

Onyekachi Ifudu, MD
Assistant Professor of Medicine
Director, Ambulatory and Inpatient
    Dialysis
SUNY Health Science Center at Brooklyn
Brooklyn, NY, USA

Carl M. Kjellstrand, MD, PhD, FACP
Professor of Medicine and Bioethics
Universtiy of Alberta Hospital
Edmonton, Canada

Edmund G. Lowrie, MD
President
National Medical Care, Inc.
Waltham, MA, USA

Andrew P. Lundin III, MD
Clinical Professor of Medicine
SUNY Health Science Center at Brooklyn
Director, Ambulatory Dialysis
Kings Country Hospital Center
Brooklyn, NY, USA

Netar P. Mallick, MD
Professor of Medicine
Department of Renal and General
   Medicine
Manchester Royal Infirmary
Manchester, UK

Fumiaki Marumo, MD
Professor and Chairman
Second Department of Internal Medicine
Tokyo Medical and Dental University
Tokyo, Japan

Friedrich K. Port, MD, MS, FACP
Director, Michigan Kidney Registry
Professor of Medicine and Epidemiology
University of Michigan
Ann Arbor, MI, USA

A.E.G. Raine, DPhil, FRCP
Professor of Renal Medicine
St. Bartholomew's Medical College
London, UK

T.K.S. Rao, MD
Professor of Medicine
SUNY Health Science Center at Brooklyn
Director, Inpatient Dialysis
Kings County Hospital Center
Brooklyn, NY, USA

Ann Sealey, RN
Dialysis Nurse
SUNY Health Science Center at Brooklyn
Kings County Hospital Center
Brooklyn, NY, USA

Stanley Shaldon, MD
Professor of Medicine
Department of Nephrology
University Hospital
Nîmes, France

Introduction to the final challenge

Life without kidneys, a marvel of our times, is now a matter of fact. This book addresses by far the most important issues about that fact – the length of such a life and what factors determine it. Considerable variability permeates this corner of our global village, there is substantial disagreement among experts and not inconsiderable frustration. Shortened dialysis times, reuse, urea kinetic modelling, patient selection, patient nutrition, what is adequate, what is optimum, how reliable are international mortality comparisons? Big issues loom and need resolution. The experts whose chapters are included here are predominantly clear analytic minds. A number are also restless souls with a passion to see optimization of the quality and quantity of life without kidneys. It is therefore an important book. It is also an unusual book: polemical at times. Eli Friedman, who saw fit to call the group together at a symposium, makes some compelling observations in Chapter 2. These remarks remain equally compelling when read as an epilogue.

Reflecting on the ingenuity of this century's search to master the inscrutable subtlety of the kidney, the epochal event since Homer Smith was the advent of ESRD therapy. It is true that the vista unfolded by Homer Smith's physiologic investigations unleashed an explosion of subsequent discoveries unparalleled in the elegance of their complexity by any other organ system, surpassing the dreams of Claude Bernard and, as of today, showing no signs of plateauing. Yet a paradox emerged: none of these discoveries is quite as remarkable as the fact that we can get along quite well without kidneys. ESRD therapy can do the job instead. That was demonstrated (if not universally accepted) more than 30 years ago. Today, when we talk of life without kidneys it is not uncommon to talk in decades. Advances have been dramatic. Machinery is very safe, vascular access is much more durable, recombinant erythropoietin is on prescription. But the most fundamental philosophical question of those early pioneering years remains the dominant practical question of today: what constitutes adequate dialysis? Indeed, the most basic of all questions in the fields of outcomes and effectiveness research, mortality and how to do something about it, has come to occupy center-stage amongst the leaders

E. A. Friedman (ed.), Death on Hemodialysis, ix–xiii.
© 1994 *Kluwer Academic Publishers.*

in the field of ESRD research; the unanswered enigma. Thirty years have gone by and now we are asking, this book is asking: Dialysis mortality, preventable or inevitable? The brave dialyzing nephrologists of the early years, often scoffed at by the disciples of the Homer Smith aftermath, yet who contributed to the solutions of so many other issues surrounding ESRD therapy, may sound perplexed, perhaps angry, that this question should be so shrouded in confusion today. At superficial glance, it sounds like we have come full circle. But this is not so. We have come to tackle the final challenge – the challenge of today's investigative clinical nephrologist, to make life without kidneys, in quality and quantity, no different from life with kidneys. This book is the introduction to that final challenge: it defines the issues and problems which now must be brought to resolution: the optimum dialysis prescription. What is adequate dialysis is an important question. It is, however, the question for the Third World. What is optimum dialysis is the question for the US. Europe and Japan must also face this issue from their perspectives.

Anyone who has frequently flown into the metropolis where these proceedings took place will likely have experienced an occasion when airport landing was delayed due to air traffic congestion; perhaps an extra hour or even half hour in an airplane seat. That's enough to appreciate what it must be like to be released from the dialysis seat half an hour or more earlier. News of shortened dialysis time can be epiphanic for a patient. Provided, of course that it does not increase his mortality. Robert Barth in a proceeding chapter implies however, that it does. "Big trouble in a small package" is how he encapsulates his analysis of available data: the blood flow rates and clearance requirements theoretically needed for optimum dialysis exceed what is being achieved in everyday reality in units practicing short dialysis. Technical limitations prevent goal congruence between what the patient receives and what the physician prescribes. Sensitized to the potential economic incentives for shortened dialysis time, Barth's perspective on life without kidneys does not rank too highly the issue of less time in the dialysis seat. But looking beyond the US, to paraphrase Carl Kjellstrand, could not several Western countries, instead of bragging about an extra year or so of survival, start to dramatically increase the number of patients offered ESRD therapy, even if it means incorporating such cost effective measures as shortened dialysis time under conditions of maximized blood flow and dialyzer surface area? After all, the current European median for patients gaining access to ESRD therapy is scarcely 25% of that in the US! Without concessions to cost cutting, Geoffrey Berlyne, whose pen played a previous role in goading the British NHS for its denial of ESRD therapy to many of its citizens, sees much room for further improvement in reducing the prevalence of "uremicide" in the UK.

Dialysis reuse is another cost-cutter. But Stanley Shaldon concludes unequivocally that it is a killer of ESRD patients. He attributes to it a major role in the recent report by Philip Held, expanded on in this volume, of higher dialysis mortality in the US compared to Europe and Japan, even after statistical correction for case mix and other relevant variables. John Bower heartily agrees. Dismissing the "first use syndrome" as a "straw man" and emphasizing the extensive *M. chelonei* outbreak that occurred in a reusing center, he sees the profit motive as the driving force for reuse and a definite source of preventable mortality. Yet, Christopher Blaggs report of 25 years of safe reuse brings attention to an aspect that must in part offset the economic driving force theory: the opposition of the manufacturing branch of the dialysis industry. Reuse is not good for sales. Blagg also estimated the global savings in environmental load of non biodegradable material resulting from reuse. Furthermore Allen Collin's analysis implies that the outbreak of *M. chelonei* is not an indictment of the principle of reuse but rather of its malpractice. And more importantly, applying the principles of utilitarian ethics and some calculations of US and European data, Kjellstrand posits a cogent hypothetical question: whether it is preferable to dialyze 1075 patients for five years or 480 patients for 10 years? The landmark publication of Gotch and colleagues, launching kinetic modelling as a tool for prescribing and monitoring hemodialysis, is still a topic for further elucidation. The theoretical and practical limitations of Kt/V, as outlined by Hans Gurland, raise the serious question as to how use of it, or some derivative of it, has become a virtual requirement for reimbursement for ESRD therapy in the US, while being largely ignored even as a useful adjunct throughout most of Europe. A model is just a model. Dialysizing by numbers can give a false sense of security. Nietzsche is surely right that simplification is falsification. No doubt kinetic modelling is a remarkable conceptual advance. It is a useful adjuvant. It is worthy of further study and investigation. As currently used it should not be the gold standard for adequate, not to mention, optimum dialysis.

All of the above, and more besides, have been incriminated as a consequence of a report which must have had a significant influence in bringing this symposium into existence, namely, Held's important survival studies which concluded that the US was trailing other advanced nations in this regard. Serious reservation must nonetheless be cast over international comparisons at the present time. Witness the far fewer patients to whom ESRD therapy is available in Europe, with the inevitable exclusion of the older and sicker, including many diabetics, and the relative rarity of transplantation in Japan, keeping the youngest and healthiest on hemodialysis with consequential improvement in the overall survival statistics of this therapeutic modality. Cox's proportional hazards statistics and Kaplan Meier methodology, when uncritically viewed, can readily bamboozle the epidemiologically uninitiated reader. Eli Friedman, Carl Kjellstrand and a few others have 'looked twice' at placing undue faith in such complexities. Nietzsche could also take note here! As far as Japan is concerned overall life expectancy is higher than in the US in the first place, kidney disease aside. Moreover, there is need to explain the data in Marimo's report on the patterns of death on dialysis in Japan, where 'heart failure' tops the list in both ESRD registry statistics and autopsy studies. This is at variance with the US experience. Lowrie studied the relative contributions of measured variables to death among hemodialysis patients. He confirmed three important predictors: the higher the serum albumin, the urea removal rate and the serum creatinine respectively, the better the survival. The two major points of this important study are the critical value of good nutrition for prolonged survival without kidneys, and the fact that the sum of all the measured variables account for only about a quarter of the deaths. With regard to the second of these points, there are clearly heretofore overlooked variables out there, waiting to be spotted by the prepared mind, which probably have associated interventional strategies that could dramatically alter the focus of a future edition of this book. In this regard Belding Scribner's emphasis on blood pressure control as a major neglected factor affecting survival of dialysis patients, can scarcely be over-emphasized as an area in need of urgent study. With regard to the first point, the serum albumin was independently confirmed by Morrell Avram's group as a survival correlate as was also the serum cholesterol. Additionally, for reasons succinctly outlined by Raine, Barth and Ritz, the dyslipidemia of uremia as a factor in mortality is in need of further investigation including therapeutic trials. Equally important, with regard to the broad area of nutrition, data from this source are sounding more and more like a final nail in the coffin of the multicenter studies of protein-restricted diets which have received such generous federal funding during the past decade. At least with hindsight it would seem that some such funds could have been better deployed in investigating the many answerable questions which constitute the chapters of this book.

Apart from selection criteria, dialysis protocols and the measurable and as yet unidentified variables alluded to, psychosocial factors influencing patient compliance, as summarized by Rao, including intravenous drug abuse, HIV disease, homelessness and the problems of undocumented aliens are likely compounding prognostic factors. Peter Lundin is to the point in reporting that many deaths in dialysis patients are preventable.

George E. Schreiner pinpointed the remarkable fact, indeed feat, that unlike any known governmentally funded activity, the unit cost of ESRD therapy has been declining over the past 20 years, surely a cause for congratulation. That new units are still opening as this book goes to press, indicates that the profit margin has not yet been eroded even if a critical stage is not too much further down the road. It doesn't take an epidemiologist to discern that large amounts of money have been made off the ESRD program, especially in its early days. Could some have been cycled back for use in furthering the quest for answers we seek, now that there is less money to go around? Federal monies that supported elegant physiologic investigations stemming from the Homer Smith tradition have been less available for ESRD research of recent decades. Has that kept us behind the curve in acquiring the outcome and effectiveness knowledge we now need? Were this not the case, would this book be less polemical? Or do polemics activate the political system? Here let us acknowledge an area where the nephrology world misled the politicians, when arguing on the floor of Congress for funding for the ESRD program in the first place: an overoptimistic view of its rehabilitative outcome was portrayed. In terms of functional status and income generating capacity, Gutman showed, a decade later, that the performance of ESRD patients was well below earlier predictions. Onyekachi Ifudu *et al.*, another decade down the road, now show how much further we have fallen below expectations with only 10% of the maintenance dialysis patients in this series gainfully employed outside the home. Sadly, the dominant reason is unchanged: fear of forfeiture of medical benefits and disability rating. The dead hand of bureaucracy! Doubtlessly the best functional and vocational rehabilitation that the ESRD program attained was with home hemodialysis patients. While acknowledging the role of patient selection, Barbara Delano's suggestion of resuscitating this therapeutic modality should not go unheard. Nor Friedrich Port's emphasis on CAPD.

Eli Friedman has looked at the big picture through a somewhat different prism. His assessment of the data reported by the National Academy of Medicine is that the mortality of dialysis patients is not increasing despite a plethora of statements to the contrary. Moreover his own evaluation of all available data lead him to the conclusion that the whole scare regarding a progressively rising death rate for hemodialysis patients in the US is erroneous, a misreading of statistics. Does this mean a call for complacency? I don't read him that way. However, rather than overfocussing on European or Japanese benchmarks where comparisons are not always readily interpretable, we in the US should retake the lead and invite all to join as we accelerate the search for the grail of optimum dialysis. It appeared for a while as if ESRD research had reached a plateau. But this is not so. Rather, as the proceeding chapters indicate, we are on a spring board. Ulysses said it right in Tennyson's poem, "much work of noble note may yet be done".

E. BOURKE, MD
Professor of Medicine
Vice-Chairman, Department of Medicine,
State University of New York,
Health Science Center at Brooklyn
Chief, Medical Service Veterans,
administration Medical Center Brooklyn

CHAPTER 1

Death on hemodialysis: preventable or inevitable?

ELI A. FRIEDMAN

> "Where shall I begin, please your Majesty? he asked.
> "Begin at the beginning," the King said, gravely, "and go on till you come to the end: then stop."
> (Lewis Carroll, *Alice's Adventures in Wonderland*)

American medical ingenuity devised and clinically established four satisfactory regimens for life prolongation in irreversible renal failure: kidney transplantation, maintenance hemodialysis, continuous ambulatory peritoneal dialysis (CAPD), hemofiltration. Under a capitalist system of health care delivery, the United States has continuously expanded the incidence rate of new patients begun on end-stage renal disease (ESRD) treatment, remaining continuously in first place among industrialized nations. In 1990, for example, the US started 182 per million new ESRD patients while the rate in Japan was 149 per million and the rates in France, Germany, and the United Kingdom were less than 80 per million [1]. By the late 1980s, however, criticism of the American ESRD system was raised both within and outside of the United States focusing on outcome of ESRD treatment as correlates of level of government funding and/or physician avarice causing perilous alteration of the dialysis prescription.

A key complaint against the American ESRD program – and American nephrologists – is that the death rate on hemodialysis has been and continues to increase out of proportion to any change in patient mix, reflecting a greater proportion of diabetics or old people. Additionally, it is alleged, the reason for the rising death rate is a merciless reduction in federal reimbursement for dialysis care to a level which forced nephrologists to practice two harmful practices: unsafe, short hemodialyses, and dialyzer reuse. It cannot be contested that there has been a reduction in payment for each hemodialysis – which, when measured in constant dollars – amounts to a decrease from $138 in 1974 to $54 in 1991 (Fig. 1).

Hull, as spokesperson for those American nephrologists who are critical of federal cost-containment policies states: "Cost-containment efforts have

E. A. Friedman (ed.), Death on Hemodialysis, 1–11.
© 1994 *Kluwer Academic Publishers.*

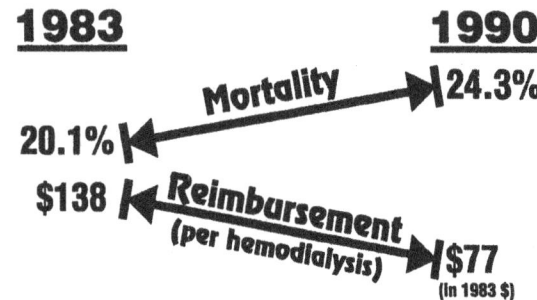

Fig. 1. Representative of several reports of the time, Berger and Lowrie accept and repeat the error in fact that there has been a sharp rise in annual hemodialysis mortality in the US (JAMA 1991; 265: 901–910). As depicted in Figs. 2 and 3, there has been no increase in US mortality though a continuing change in case mix has occurred. Older, sicker patients have been accepted each year for the past 20 years.

resulted in progressive reductions in reimbursement proved by Medicare to both physicians and dialysis centers.... It is likely that these reimbursement restrictions have negatively impacted the level of patient care; both mortality and morbidity rates in patients receiving chronic dialysis are increasing in the United States. This is a significant cause for concern, particularly as the mortality rates in other industrialized countries began much lower than the US rate and have continued to decline despite adding older and presumably sicker patients" [2]. Held *et al.* used a Cox proportional hazards model (multivariate) to detect a linkage between reduction in reimbursement and 3-year patient survival for 14,807 new hemodialysis patients who started dialysis in 1984 [3]. While lower payments were associated with a shift in unit personnel from registered nurses to practical nurses and technicians: "There was no statistically significant relationship between the level of staffing in the dialysis unit or the percent of staff who were RNs and 3-year patient survival." Kjellstrand, in a scathing attack on short dialysis charged: "There are many reasons to shorten dialysis, none of them medical" [4]. Reviewing survival data from the same era, Shaldon concluded: "Recent data presented to the FDA by the NIH and the Urban Institute suggest that reuse may indeed be a factor in explaining the difference in survival data between the United States and the rest of the civilized world" [5].

There thus arose four interrelated indictments against the American way of delivering maintenance hemodialysis for ESRD (Table 1):

On April 26, 1993, a conference sponsored by the International Society for Artificial Organs (ISAO) was held in Brooklyn, New York to examine the grave allegations enumerated in Table 1. While the issues are complex, and some statistical methods are limited in comprehension to a few experts, it was possible to extract inferences which are likely to mature into truths.

Table 1. Alleged deficiencies in US delivery of maintenance hemodialysis

1.	US has a progressively rising death rate for standard maintenance hemodialysis.
2.	Short hemodialysis promotes excess mortality.
3.	Hemodialyzer reuse is dangerous and promotes excess mortality.
4.	Compared with Europe or Japan, US maintenance hemodialysis has excess mortality.

The chapters which follow are the product of participants at the meeting, sometimes expounding views at extreme variance with each other.

As conference organizer, I was afforded the vantage position of referee without an ox to be gored. This program's affiliated hemodialysis units are *not for profit*, do not champion short treatment times, and do not practice hemodialyzer reuse. Surprisingly, though the initial and sustained attacks on the system provoked an uneasy, subjective feeling that injustice was being been done to American ESRD patients, careful examination of the available evidence does not support such a dark interpretation of the recent relationship between the government and renal providers of care. Firstly, it is impossible to counter the argument – independently validated as true by the author – that the commercial market price for *for profit* hemodialysis facilities is rising, or at worst, holding constant. Among colleagues throughout the US, there is pressure, in some instances, a rush, to open new hemodialysis facilities, *for profit*. How can it be, then, that the federal reimbursement rate had fallen below the level necessary for dialysis facilities to remain financially solvent? Physician-owned corporations questing for new earning opportunities, based on federal government reimbursement standards, do not aggressively pursue businesses which are doomed to lose money for any reason, let alone a fundamental funding limitation imposed by the federal government.

The four points raised in Table 1 will now be addressed in order.

1.   The US has a progressively rising death rate for standard maintenance hemodialysis

It may be difficult to discover the origin of a myth – in this instance, the rumor that the death rate of US, dialysis patients is increasing. This is not true. Study of the USRDS published annual reports for the past three years indicates that rather than a progressive decline, there actually has been a slow but unquestionable improvement in one-year survival on dialysis. Actually, all data in the USRDS suffers from the flaw that survival times and all other treatment events begin on the 91st day of ESRD therapy, a time when funding is first assumed. Thus, when detailing first-year survival, what is being described is survival from the 91st day to 1 year plus 90 days. Regard Figs. 2 and 3, derived from data supplied by the USRDS, which make it ineluctably clear that over the decade from 1980 to 1990, mortality has not increased for the whole US ESRD cohort or its component subsets. Indeed, for the youngest age groups and for diabetics, survival has progressively improved.

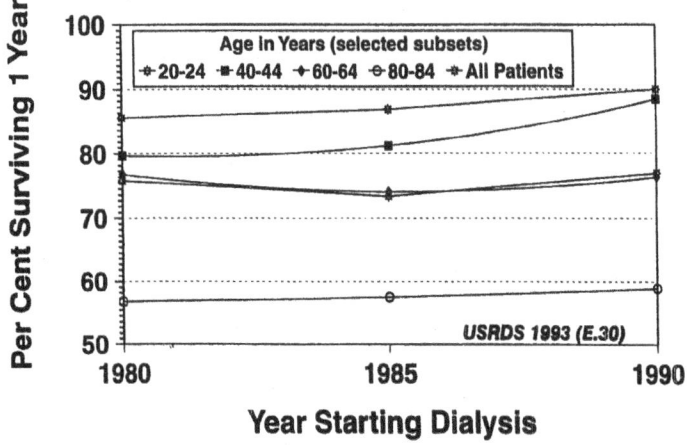

Fig. 2.   Selected age subsets of total US ESRD population. Survival after one year and 91 days on dialysis in 1980, 1985, and 1990. Note the overall survival for all ESRD patients is given and has risen slightly over the decade. Source: USRDS 1993 Report.

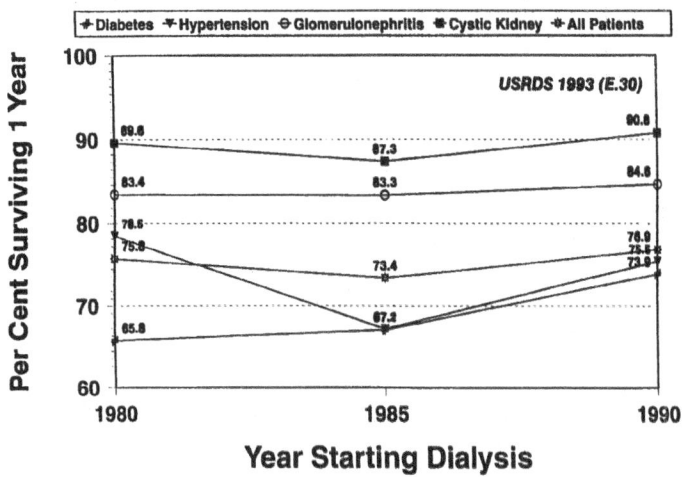

Fig. 3.   Selected renal diagnosis subsets of total US ESRD population. Survival after one year and 91 days on dialysis in 1980, 1985, and 1990. Note the overall survival for all ESRD patients is given and has risen slightly over the decade. Source: USRDS 1993 Report.

If the preceding inference is correct, the question leaping immediately to the foreground is: Where did the assertion that US dialysis death rates were rising originate? In all probability, a slight rise in the death rate of some subsets of patients from 1980 to 1983 was extrapolated and used as a basis for generalization beyond the limits of supporting data.

Because of the serious consequences of the charge that inadequate government reimbursement rates were responsible for a greater 'die off' of dialysis patients, the National Academy of Medicine conducted a full fledged evaluation of the ESRD program. After two years of review, including interviews with legislators, physicians, health administrators, and economists, this study concluded that: "Gross mortality has been increasing, but age-adjusted and diagnosis-adjusted mortality have been quite stable. This implies that the increasing age and complexity of the patient population may account for much of the observed increase in mortality. However, adjustment for ESRD patient complexity is somewhat crude at present, being limited to standardization for the effects of patient age, gender, race, and primary diagnoses. More refined means to adjust for patient complexity may be needed to detect significant mortality changes among subgroups of the patient population" [6].

Reviewing selected mortality data and under the attack of several articulate nephrologists, a battered National Academy of Medicine committee wavered in its assessment of US handling of dialysis reimbursement: "The committee believes that these data suggest the possibility that decreases in reimbursement may have led to increases in mortality indirectly via an economic incentive to shorten treatment times, which in turn led to increased mortality" [7]. It is the author's conclusion that: *Evidence does not justify the allegation that the mortality of patients receiving hemodialysis treatments in the US is rising.*

2. Short hemodialysis promotes excess mortality

Starting with the National Cooperative Dialysis Study performed over a decade ago [8], the relationship between inordinate short dialysis and increased morbidity has been recognized. On one side, the best-reported long-term dialysis results – 43% survival at 20 years – is attributed to the Tassin unit in France [9] which delivers long dialysis (24 or more hours per week). Without antihypertensives or erythropoietin, these "unselected" French patients appear to attain the best possible outcome. As practiced by Charra *et al.* "Adequate dialysis cannot be reduced to numbers: it should include both sufficient small- and middle-molecule diffusion and ultrafiltration with arterial pressure control without need for anti-hypertensive medication" [10].

By contrast, proponents of short hemodialsyis treatment schedules "approximately three 3-hour treatments per week," pointed to their high survival rates (91% at 1 year, 60% at 10 years) to underscore their contention that such short dialysis "may be safely applied for at least 9 years" [11]. More recent support for the concept of safe, short hemodialysis, especially when coupled with hi-flux membranes and high blood flow rates is present in reports elsewhere in this volume.

Issuing a clarion call to halt unnecessary deaths on US, hemodialysis programs, Held *et al.* investigated the relationship of duration of each dialysis treatment to 3-year mortality in a sample of 600 dialysis patients from 36 dialysis units [12]. These workers, using the Cox model, adjusted for other patient and dialysis unit covariates, found that "duration of the dialysis procedure is an important element in determining patient mortality as one of the factors determining the adequacy of dialysis." Patients receiving an average

Table 2. Possible explanations for high US dialysis mortality

1.	AIDS patients.
2.	Narcotics abusers.
3.	Homeless and other sociopathic patients.
4.	Illegal immigrants with poor nutrition and co-morbid disorders.
5.	Enrollment of 'marginal' patients refused elsewhere (malignancy, senility, psychosis, mental deficiency).
6.	There is no higher mortality when proper subsets are compared.

dialysis treatment of less than 3.5 hours had a relative mortality risk of 1.17 to 2.18 compared with those whose treatments were longer than 3.5 hours. An editorial in the same issue of JAMA agreed with the conclusions of Held *et al.* and again raised the issue of whether reductions in funding were the root cause for shorter dialyses which escalated death rate [13].

While the length of dialysis debate is ongoing, it should be recalled that the origin of concern over shortening dialysis was the purported increasing death rate which is not increasing at all. In the author's view, dialysis duration should be determined clinically on the basis of patient well being, maintenance of muscle mass, avoidance of hypertensive medications, and minimized requirement for erythropoietin. Based on personal observation, in dialysis units throughout the world, it seems likely that the majority of dialysis patients presently are underdialyzed. A combination of variables leads to this sorry state, of which, too short a dialysis time, is an important variable. With some exceptions, however, underdialysis appeared as prevalent in Japan, Italy, Germany and Israel as in the US. Of course, the subjective, impressionistic kind of observations which led the author to this position do not reflect a scientific international survey of adequacy of dialysis.

3.   Hemodialyzer reuse is dangerous and promotes excess mortality

From the patient's perspective, reuse of hemodialysis cartridges is of no benefit. Nephrologists attempting to justify what amounts to an economy-based decision on patient care were inventive with rationalizations of why something obviously adding to the risk of a hemodialysis treatment might be good for patients. For example, previously, avoidance of a nebulous, *first-use syndrome* consisting of back and/or chest pain with or without hypotension, was suggested as grounds for reusing dialyzer cartridges. When studied prospectively, however, "the incidence of chest pain and back pain was no longer greater during first use than during reuse" [14]. Cheung *et al.* also concluded that: "maintenance hemodialysis with reused cellulose acetate membrane dialyzers processed with hydrogen peroxide and peroxyacetic acid was not associated with more or fewer subjective symptoms than dailies with new dialyzers" [15].

On the other side of the analysis, hemodialyzer reuse brings significant risk of microbial contamination and exposure to residual quantities of sterilants

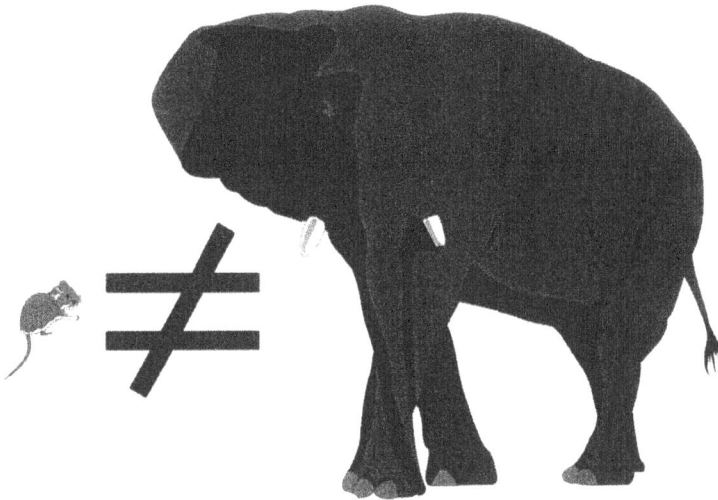

Fig. 4. Even with statistical adjustment for size and weight, an elephant and a mouse cannot be considered as equivalent when comparing subjects or groups of subjects. Younger, healthier Europeans are not equivalent to older, sicker Americans when comparing annual survival on hemodialysis. Other factors contribute to differences in American and European dialysis subsets, especially, the exclusion policies in Europe which amount to ESRD incidence rates of one-half or less that of the US.

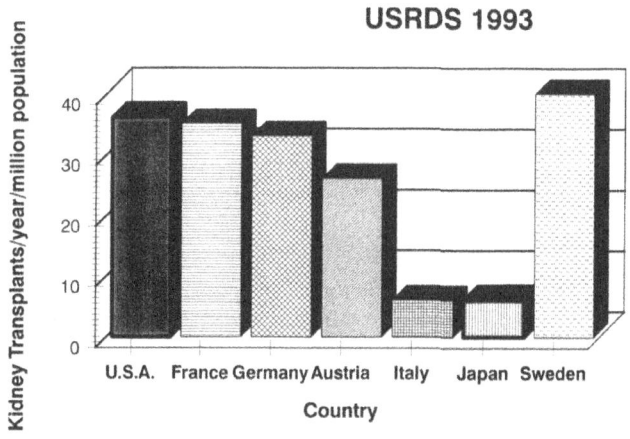

Fig. 5. Kidney transplant rate in 1990 (selected countries: USRDS 1993). Japan accepts fewer patients for renal transplantation. This means that the prime group usually referred for a renal transplant, the young, relatively healthy patient without extrarenal disease is retained on maintenance hemodialysis. Improvement in dialysis survival is a necessary consequence. This and other variables may account for US – Japanese disparity in dialysis mortality.

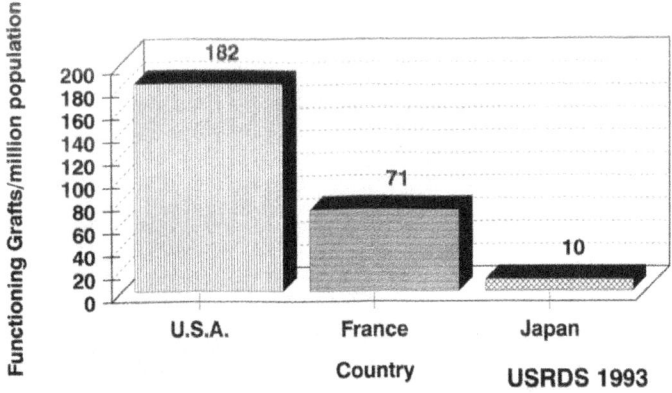

Fig. 6. Functioning kidney transplant rate in 1990 (USRDS 1993). While present acceptance rate for renal transplants have improved in Europe, note that France, has a prevalence of transplant recipients that is only 39% the US rate. This means that patients who would have received a transplant in the US are retained on dialysis in France. Couple this reality with the low acceptance rate for ESRD in France and a picture emerges of either extensive underprovision of uremia therapy in France or a different attack rate (incidence) for the same disease in France than the US. Statistical adjustments will not nullify this variable. The question of why? remains open.

as well as any denaturation products of membrane change which may have been produced. The author is aware of several unreported incidents in which patient deaths followed dialysis with an improperly prepared, reused dialyzer. Shaldon states without equivocation that: "The total failure to guarantee sterility has resulted in deaths directly attributable to reuse. A moratorium on reuse is suggested" [16]. Stragier describes an explosion due to improperly mixed disinfecting solution [17]. More usually, however, esthetic and scientific objections to application of reused dialyzers are less calmly recognized or countered. Personal observation of dialyzers reused for 60 or more times has led the author to the position that reuse of dialyzers should not be accepted until all other means of fiscal restraint have been introduced. One Canadian 'cost-minimization analysis' indicated that reusing a dialyzer four times (five uses) might save up to $3,629 (Canadian dollars) per patient yearly or $5.8 to $8.9 million per year [18]. Weighing the pros and cons of hemodialyzer reuse, the National Kidney Foundation found that under optimal conditions, dialyzers could be reused safely, but that "patients should have the right to refuse application of a reused dialyzer" [19].

As was contended for shortened dialysis times, dialyzer reuse cannot be blamed for a rise in US mortality on maintenance hemodialysis because there has been no such increase. Dialyzer reuse should be viewed as an economic measure, introducing hazard to patients, which may nevertheless prove necessary to permit treatment of all suitable patients with the funding provided by government.

4.   Compared with Europe or Japan, US maintenance hemodialysis has excess mortality

Many workers believe this thesis to be established and no longer debatable. For example, the report of Levin *et al.* accepts the difference in death rates as increasing: "With recent startling statistics showing an increase in mortality risk of dialysis patients in the United States compared to other countries, managers and practitioners have been motivated to carefully examine not only the dialysis prescription, but what is actually delivered to the patient" [20]. In the same vein, Held *et al* state as a given that: "Controlling for age and diabetes, patients with end-stage renal disease in Europe generally have better rates of survival that do ESRD patients in the US" [21]. A substantially greater amount of dialysis was provided in Europe, these workers conclude, because of use of larger surface area dialyzers and longer hemodialysis treatments.

The author remains unconvinced – with an open mind – that the mortality on dialysis is greater in the US than in Japan or Europe. There is no doubt that crude (unadjusted) death rates are higher in the US. The enormous question of how to construct equivalent subsets of ESRD patients for comparison of outcome persists and must dominate the inquiry.

In 1957, the median age of newly treated US ESRD patients–60 years-was highest of all countries monitored by the USRDS [22]. By comparison, the median age of incident Japanese ESRD patients was 53 years, while those starting treatment in the UK had a median age of 54 years. That increasingly older patients are being accepted in the US is evident from the rise in median age of incident ESRD patients to 62 years in 1990. The reader may best appreciate the inequity of comparing unequal groups by reviewing reports of rehabilitation or return to employment in which ESRD patients treated by dialysis are contrasted with those given a renal transplant. Differences of as much as 20 years between median age in the two groups preclude any true comparison, even by use of the Cox proportional hazards statistical approach. As shown in Fig.4, which extrudes the discussion to the absurd, one cannot consider a mouse equivalent to an elephant, just by making adjustment for disparity in size and weight.

There are major differences in how ESRD populations are selected in the US, Europe, and Japan. Kjellstrand, elsewhere in this text, explores this contention fully. One need note only the relative incidence rates for new ESRD patients in Europe and the US, to come to the conclusion that either ESRD has a much lower incidence in Europe, or Europe is excluding patients who reasonably might otherwise be treated. In this context, when the Tassin group (detailed above) reports outstanding survival in an unselected population, either they do not recognize that a selection process has been utilized, or it is three times healthier (for the kidneys) to live in France than in the US.

Likewise, in terms of Japanese acceptance to ESRD programs, there is both a marked deficiency in proffering a transplant (Fig. 5) which cumulatively means retention of young, healthier patients on dialysis and a restricted pool of surviving transplant recipients (Fig. 6). When Held *et al.* elsewhere in these pages detects a sharp difference in survival for one year between Japanese and Americans, it has not been established to the author's satisfaction that the dissimilarity results from comparing different risk groups.

The American approach to and delivery of uremia therapy must be questioned, evaluated, and reevaluated continuously. Caution is warranted, however, in coming to a judgment before-the-fact. It was the Queen of Hearts in *Alice's Adventures in Wonderland* who delivered Lewis Carroll's apt warning when proclaiming: "Off with his head! No! No! Sentence first – verdict afterwards!"

References

1. US Renal Data System, USRDS 1993 Annual Data Report, The National Institutes of Health, National Institute of Diabetes and Digestive and Kidney Diseases, Bethesda, MD, March 1993.
2. Hull AR. Impact of reimbursement regulations on patient management. Am J Kidney Dis 1992; 20 (1 Suppl 1): 8–11.
3. Held PJ, Garcia JR, Pauly MV, Cahn. Price of dialysis, unit staffing, and length of dialysis treatments. Am J Kidney Dis 1990; 15: 441–450.
4. Kjellstrand CM. Short dialysis increases morbidity and mortality. Contrib Nephrol 1985; 44: 65–67.
5. Shaldon S. Dialyzer reuse: A practice that should be abandoned. Seminars Dialysis 1993; 6: 11–12.
6. Rettig RA and Levinsky NG, editors. *Kidney Failure and the Federal government*. Washington, DC: National Academy Press, 1991; 215.
7. Rettig RA and Levinsky NG, editors. *Kidney Failure and the Federal Government*. Washington, DC: National Academy Press, 1991; 214.
8. Lowrie EG, Teehan BP. Principles of prescribing dialysis therapy: implementing recommendations from the National Cooperative Dialysis Study. Kidney Int Suppl 1983; 13: S113–S122.
9. Charra B, Calemard E, Ruffet M, Chazot C, Terrat JC, Vanel T, Laurent G. Survival as an index of adequacy of dialysis. Kidney Int 1992; 41: 1286–1291.
10. Charra B, Calemard E, Chazot C, Terrat JC, Vanel T, Ruffet M, Laurent G. Dose of dialysis, what index? Blood Purif 1992; 10: 13–21.
11. Wauters JP, Bercini-Pansiot S, Gilliard N, Stauffer JC. Short hemodialysis: long-term mortality and morbidity. Artif Organs 1986; 10: 182–184.
12. Held PJ, Levin NW, BovbJerg RR, Pauly MV, Diamond LH. Mortality and duration of hemodialysis treatment. JAMA 1991; 265: 861–875.
13. Berger EE, Lowrie EG. Mortality and the length of dialysis. JAMA 1991; 265: 909–910.
14. Charoenpanich R, Pollak VE, Kant KS, Robson MD, Cathey M. Effect of first and subsequent use of hemodialyzers on patient well being: the rise and fall of a syndrome associated with new dialyzer use. Artif Organs 1987; 11: 123–127.
15. Cheung AK, Dalpias D, Emmerson R, Leypoldt JK. A prospective study on intradialytic symptoms associated with reuse of hemodialyzers. Am J Nephrol 1991; 11: 397–401.
16. Shaldon S. Unanswered questions pertaining to dialysis adequacy in 1992. Kidney Int Suppl 1993; 41: S274–S277.
17. Stragier A. ANNA J Hazards with disinfecting agents in renal units! ANNA J 1992; 87: 41–43.
18. Baris E, McGregor M. The reuse of hemodialyzers: an assessment of safety and potential savings. Can Med Assoc J 1993; 148: 175–183.
19. National Kidney Foundation report on dialyzer reuse. Am J Kidney Dis 1988; 11: 1–6.

20. Levin N, Gotch F, Bednar B, Gallagher N, Peterson G, Bednar B. Kinetics and quality assurance: prescription therapy through kinetic modeling. ANNA J 1991; 18: 269–290.
21. Held PJ, Blagg CR, Liska DW, Port FK, Hakim R, Levin N. The dose of hemodialysis according to dialysis prescription in Europe and the United States. Kidney Int Suppl 1992; 38: S16–S21.
22. US Renal Data System, USRDS 1990 Annual Data Report, The National Institutes of Health, National Institute of Diabetes and Digestive and Kidney Disease, Bethesda, MD, August 1990.

CHAPTER 2

Survival of middle-aged dialysis patients in Japan and the US, 1988–89

PHILIP J. HELD, TAKASHI AKIBA, NAOKO S. STEARNS,
FUMIAKI MARUMO, MARC N. TURENNE, KENJI MAEDA and
FRIEDRICH K. PORT

Introduction

Previous comparisons of the survival of end-stage renal disease (ESRD) patients in the US with Europe and Japan indicated worse survival outcomes for the US, with adjustment for differences in age and diabetes [1]. A similar set of survival comparisons between Japan and the US was presented at a recent conference in New York [2] (April 26, 1993) for a newer cohort of incident patients treated with continuous ambulatory peritoneal dialysis (CAPD) and hemodialysis (HD). This report summarizes the results of those across-country comparisons, with added consideration given to the expected survival of dialysis patients compared to the expected survival of the general population in both societies.

Survival comparisons were limited to incident dialysis patients between the ages of 45 and 64 years at onset of ESRD. This age group represents a substantial proportion of the ESRD population in both countries, yet is less likely to receive a kidney transplant than younger age groups in the US [3]. Analyses of this middle-aged group of patients rather than younger patients may reduce the effects of healthier US patients being selected for kidney transplantation, a procedure that is seldom done in Japan [4]. As with a previous study comparing Japan with the US [1], Japanese survival estimates were directly standardized to the US population, in this case by age, gender, diabetic status, and treatment modality (CAPD, HD). The ratio of the life expectancy of dialysis patients divided by the life expectancy of the general population was also compared by country, thereby controlling for the mortality effects of differences in the non-ESRD populations. There may, however, be other differences between Japan and the US with regard to various demographic and comorbid risk factors and the adequacy of dialysis treatments, factors which may affect survival comparisons reported in the current study.

E. A. Friedman (ed.), Death on Hemodialysis, 13–23.
© 1994 *Kluwer Academic Publishers.*

Methods and data

Sources of data

The analysis of one- and two-year survival probabilities was based on 1989 incident dialysis patients for the age groups 45 to 54 and 55 to 64 in Japan ($n = 7,461$) and 1988 incident dialysis patients of the same age cohorts in the US ($n = 10,783$). The Japanese data were obtained from the Japanese Society for Dialysis Therapy [5]. The US data were obtained from the US Department of Health and Human Services, Health Care Financing Administration Program Medical Management and Information System, May 1992 [6].

Analysis methods

The survival probabilities of the Japanese and US dialysis patients were computed in a similar manner using the Kaplan-Meier (K-M) method [7]. The K-M product-limit estimate is consistent in dealing with censored data [8]. The K-M estimates of survival probabilities [9] for the US were implemented in the SAS LIFETEST procedure and Greenwood's formula.

The 1989 incident patients in Japan were defined as those who started renal replacement therapy in 1989. They were censored at transplant or at the end of follow-up of one and two years since the onset of ESRD. As for the US patients, the 1988 incident cohorts were defined as those starting ESRD therapy in 1988, surviving at least 90 days after the ESRD therapy, and not receiving a transplant in the first 90 days. Therefore, the one year survival probability for the US dialysis patients was estimated from day 91 to one year plus 90 days. Similarly, the two year survival probability was based on the interval from day 91 to two years plus 90 days. This 90 day restriction is necessary to account for the fact that many patients in the US under age 65 do not become eligible for Medicare until day 91 and thus are incompletely captured in the US database, which includes only Medicare patients.

When the USRDS survival probabilities of the 0–12 month time period were compared with the 3–15 month time period for the 1987–1988 incident Medicare patients (age 65–69) for whom the USRDS reports reasonably complete data, it was shown that the survival probabilities during months 3–15 were higher than those during months 0–12 [10]. To correct the US estimates in this paper for the absence of survival data for the first three months, the estimates for the first and second year following month three were weighted by the ratio of the estimates starting day 0 to the estimates starting day 90, computed for the 1987–1988 incident Medicare patients (age 65–69).

Throughout this analysis, a direct standardization method was used to adjust the K-M survival estimates so that the comparison of the Japanese and US survival estimates are independent of the differences in distributions across these population parameters for the two societies. Direct standardization is a process which adjusts aggregate estimates (across-age groups or across-diagnoses) of one population by the relative weights of those groups in another population. Since the Japanese dialysis patients in this study were on average younger and less likely to be diabetic (these two factors contribute to higher survival) than their US counterparts, standardizing the Japanese estimates to the US distribution by these factors lowers the Japanese estimates. Thus, Japanese standardized estimates shown in this paper are lower than those in earlier reports for Japan.

The percentage difference in the survival estimates observed can be translated into a relative risk of mortality for US patients compared with Japanese patients. A relative risk is the ratio of the natural logarithm (ln) of the two survivals. For example, in comparing 95 and 90 percent survival estimates between groups A and B, a relative risk of A compared with B is computed as ln(.95)/ln(.90) = –0.05/–0.105 = 0.487. This means that group A has a 51 percent lower mortality risk than group B. Conversely, a relative risk of B compared with A is computed as ln(.90)/ln(.95) = –0.105/–0.05 = 2.05, indicating that group B has a 2.05 times greater mortality risk than group A.

An extension of a survival analysis is a comparison of expected remaining lifetimes of dialysis patients relative to those of the general population. If we assume that the death rates of dialysis patients do not change with time since first ESRD therapy, it is reasonable and practical to assume that the lifetime data follow an exponential distribution. The estimated death rate, $\hat{\lambda}$, is equal to $- \log(S(t))/t$, where $S(t)$ is a K–M survival estimate at time t(in years) since the first ESRD therapy. Then the expected remaining lifetime for dialysis patients, $\hat{t}_e$, is estimated as: $\hat{t}_e = 1/\hat{\lambda}$ [4]. The life expectancies of the general populations in Japan and the US are based on the current life table method which applies the age-specific death rates prevailing in a given period to the actual population to compute the expected remaining lifetime [11,12,13]. The age-specific death rates in 1990 were used for the 1990 population estimates to obtain the expected remaining lifetime of the general population in Japan. For the US, the age-specific death rates in 1988 were applied to the 1989 population estimates to compute the life expectancy of the general population.

Results

Table 1 provides overall characteristics of the incident cohorts aged 45 to 64 years in Japan and in the US. The distribution of US patients by age, diabetic renal diseases, gender, and treatment modality differs from that of Japanese patients. Japan has a higher proportion of incident patients in the 45–64 age group (45.8) than the US (34.2). Among patients in the current sample, a comparison of average ages in each ten-year age group for analysis (45–54 and 55–64 years) indicates Japanese patients (49.8 and 59.6 years, respectively) are slightly younger than US patients (50.4 and 60.4). The US incident patients are more likely to be diabetic than the Japanese patients; 42.0 percent in the US versus 31.9 percent in Japan. The percent of patients who

Table 1. Characteristics of incident CAPD and HD patients treated in Japan (1989) and the US (1988),[a] ages 45–64 years

Patient characteristics	Japan	US
Ages 45–64 (as % of patients of all ages)	45.8	34.2
Mean Age (years		
Ages 45–54	49.8	50.4
Ages 55–64	59.6	60.4
Percent of Patients Ages 45–64		
Diabetic	31.9	42.0
Female	37.2	47.0
CAPD	3.9	10.0
n	7,461	10,783

Sources: Japanese Society for Dialysis Therapy (JSDT); Health Care
Financing Administration (HCFA), US Department of Health and Human Services.
[a] US Medicare patients only.

are females in this study is 47.0 percent in the US, while it is 37.2 percent in Japan. Ten percent of the US patients and 3.9 percent of the Japanese patients were treated with CAPD. In summary, these estimates indicate that the Japanese middle-aged dialysis patients were younger, less likely to be diabetic or female, and the treatment modality selected was less likely to be CAPD than their US counterparts. The differences that exist between the two groups of patients, shown in the composition of age, diagnosis, gender and treatment modality, illustrate the need to adjust the survival estimates by these factors to allow comparison across the two societies.

Table 2 shows one- and two-year survival probabilities by primary diagnosis, gender, age and treatment modality for the dialysis patients in Japan and the US. The Japanese patients in every category report a higher survival than the US patients. The patients in every subgroup but one (diabetic, male, 55–64, CAPD) in Japan have one-year survival probabilities higher than 0.90. In contrast, the US patients have one-year survival probabilities between 0.65 to 0.87. Similarly for the two-year survival, the Japanese patients have a higher survival than the US patients.

The survival estimates for the middle-aged dialysis patients are presented in Fig. 1 for non-diabetic patients and Fig. 2 for diabetic patients. The Japanese survival estimates are standardized to the gender and modality distribution for the US dialysis patients.

Figure 1 shows that the non-diabetic dialysis patients in Japan survived longer than those in the US. It also indicates, not surprisingly, that the survival probabilities are higher for the younger patients in each country. The one-year

Table 2. Kaplan-Meier patient survival probabilities for incident dialysis patients in Japan (1988) and the US (1988) by primary diagnosis, gender, age, and treatment modality, ages 45–64 years

Primary diagnosis	Gender	Age at onset of ESRD	Treatment modality[a]	n		Kaplan-Meier patient survival probability			
						1 Year		2 Years	
				Japan	US	Japan	US[b]	Japan	US[b]
Non-Diabetic	Male	45–54	Hemodialysis	1,278	1,321	0.970	0.837	0.921	0.723
			CAPD	69	110	1.000	0.821	0.951	0.691
		55–64	Hemodialysis	1,638	1,899	0.933	0.754	0.832	0.621
			CAPD	57	204	0.962	0.711	0.864	0.530
	Female	45–54	Hemodialysis	910	890	0.964	0.855	0.925	0.751
			CAPD	52	127	0.980	0.874	0.959	0.718
		55–64	Hemodialysis	1,042	1,511	0.919	0.780	0.835	0.634
			CAPD	35	187	0.971	0.799	0.912	0.569
Diabetic	Male	45–54	Hemodialysis	563	807	0.950	0.753	0.837	0.594
			CAPD	25	95	0.960	0.817	0.831	0.618
		55–64	Hemodialysis	1,016	1,143	0.926	0.703	0.774	0.498
			CAPD	36	137	0.889	0.723	0.599	0.461
	Female	45–54	Hemodialysis	248	700	0.937	0.782	0.860	0.605
			CAPD	5	94	1.000	0.790	1.000	0.559
		55–64	Hemodialysis	476	1,433	0.930	0.746	0.810	0.559
			CAPD	11	125	0.909	0.647	0.649	0.395

Sources: JSDT; HCFA.

[a] Treatment modality was defined at day 90 following onset of ESRD for US patients.

[b] US patient survival starting at day 90 following ESRD onset was adjusted for the mortality of patients during the first 90 days. This was done by weighting survival estimates for the US by the ratio of (patient survival starting at day 0) / (patient survival starting at day 90) following ESRD onset for a subset of elderly patients (age 65–69) incident in 1987–88. Source: USRDS 1991 Annual Data Report, p. 32.

survival probability for the younger age group is 97 percent for the Japanese cohort and 84.5 percent for the US cohort. As for the older cohort, the one-year survival probability is 93.1 percent in Japan and 76.4 percent in the US. Similar patterns exist for the two-year survival. The proportion of patients alive is 92.6 percent in Japan and 73.2 percent in the US for the younger age group, and 83.9 percent and 62.3 percent for the older age group in Japan and the US, respectively.

To compare estimates from this study, a relative risk (RR) of mortality for the US patients compared with the Japanese patients was computed. For example, the 12.5 percent difference for the one year survival probability of the non-diabetic patients (age 45–54) corresponds to a RR of 5.53 ($\ln(0.845)/\ln(.97) = -0.168/-0.030$) for the US patients compared with the Japanese patients. Stated differently, the US dialysis patients have a five times greater mortality risk than the Japanese patients in this age and diagnostic group in the first year of ESRD therapy. When comparing the older cohort

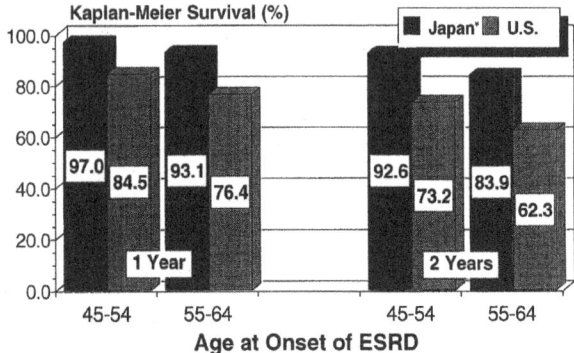

Sources: JSDT; HCFA.
*Standardized to the gender and modality (CAPD, HD) distribution for U.S.
dialysis patients. n (U.S.) = 6,249; n (Japan) = 5,081.

Fig. 1. One- and two-year survival for incident dialysis patients, Japan (1989) and the US (1988), ages 45–64, non-diabetic.

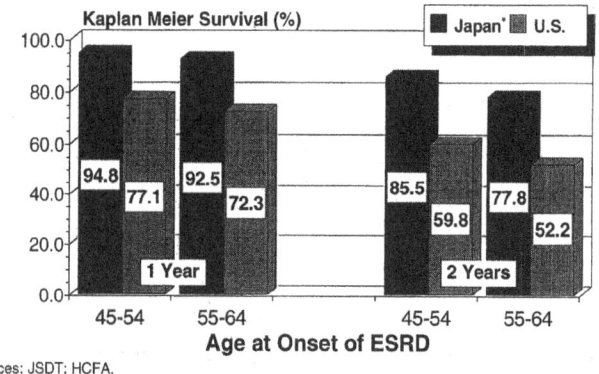

Sources: JSDT; HCFA.
*Standardized to the gender and modality (CAPD, HD) distribution for U.S.
dialysis patients. n (U.S.) = 4,534; n (Japan) = 2,380.

Fig. 2. One- and two-year survival for incident dialysis patients, Japan (1989) and the US (1988), ages 45–64, diabetic.

(age 55–64), the relative mortality risk of the US patients compared with the Japanese patients is reduced to 3.8. The same diminishing trends across two age cohorts exist for the two-year survival. The US non-diabetic patients have a 4.1 times greater mortality risk than those in Japan for the younger group, but 2.7 times for the older group. Therefore, we find that the US non-diabetic patients have a higher mortality risk than the Japanese non-diabetic patients, and is particularly true for the younger compared to the older age group and also for the one-year compared to the two-year survival.

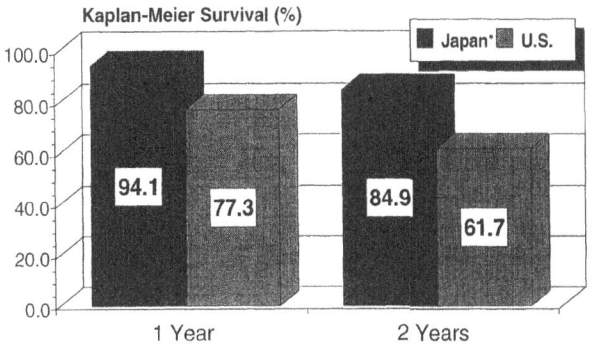

Sources: JSDT; HCFA.
*Standardized to the age, diabetes, gender and modality (CAPD, HD) distribution
for U.S. dialysis patients. n (U.S.) = 10,783; n (Japan) = 7,461.

Fig. 3. One- and two-year survival for incident dialysis patients, Japan (1989) and the US (1988), ages 45–64.

Figure 2 presents one- and two-year survival estimates for diabetic patients. As with non-diabetic patients, a decreasing survival is observed in the comparison of across-country, across-age groups and across-survival length. The Japanese and US patients show a one-year survival of 94.8 percent and 77.1 percent, respectively, for the age group 45–54. Similarly for the age group 55–64, the one-year survival probability is 92.5 percent in Japan and 72.3 percent in the US. As for the two-year survival probability, the Japanese survival for two age groups drop below 90 percent. The survival estimate is 85.5 percent in Japan compared with 59.8 percent in the US for the younger age group, while it is 77.8 percent in Japan and 52.2 percent in the US for the older age group.

The narrowing differences of the mortality risk as we compare the younger versus older age group and the one- versus two-year survival seen in the non-diabetic patients are also observed for the diabetic patients. The RRs of the US diabetic patients are 4.9 vs. 4.2 for the younger vs. older one-year survival, and 3.3 vs. 2.6 for the younger vs. older two-year survival. Even among the diabetic patients, the mortality risk of the US patients are two to four times greater than the Japanese patients, but the relative risk is higher among the younger cohort than the older cohort and higher in the one-year survival than the two-year survival. Furthermore, a comparison of the relative risks between non-diabetic and diabetic patients indicates that the mortality risks of the US patients are more pronounced for the non-diabetic group than for the diabetic group. Thus, it is clear from these estimates that the dialysis patients in Japan report a higher survival than those in the US; however, the magnitude of the differences seem to relate to the age, diagnosis and survival length being measured.

Table 3. Life expectancy for incident dialysis patients and general population in Japan and the US, ages 45–64 years

	Expected remaining lifetime (ERL), in years		
	General population	Dialysis patients	ERL ratio (%): dialysis/general
Japan (1989)[a]	27.4	12.2	44.5%
US (1988)	27.0	4.1	15.3%

Sources: JSDT; HCFA.

[a] Directly standardized to the corresponding US population according to age (5-year age groups), gender, and in the case of dialysis patients, primary cause of ESRD (diabetes, not diabetes) and treatment modality (CAPD, hemodialysis).

Figure 3 provides an overall version of survival for these two age groups in both the US and Japan. Figure 3 shows aggregate (across-age, across-gender, across-diagnosis across-modality) survival estimates for the one- and two-year survival. The Japanese estimates were adjusted by all of the aggregate factors for the US patients. The one-year survival probability is 94.1 percent in Japan and 77.3 percent in the US, and the two-year survival probability is 84.9 percent in Japan and 61.7 percent in the US.

The 16.7 percent difference for the one-year survival is translated to a RR of 4.2 for the US compared with Japan. Therefore, these estimates suggest that the US patients of the age 45–64 cohort have an adjusted mortality risk that is 4.2 times greater than that of their Japanese counterparts one year after the ESRD therapy, and 2.9 times two years after the initiation of renal replacement therapy.

Table 3 compares the life expectancy of dialysis patients and the general population in Japan and the US. The estimates for Japan are standardized to the age, gender, diagnosis and modality distribution of the US patients. The expected remaining lifetime (ERL) in years is estimated to be 12.2 years for the Japanese dialysis patients aged 45 to 64 years, while the ERL is only 4.1 years for the US dialysis patients of the same age cohort. However, the ERLs of the general populations are very close in both countries: 27.4 years for Japan and 27.0 years for the US. By expressing these estimates in terms of the ratio of the ERL of the dialysis patients to the general population, the effects of mortality differences between the non-ESRD populations in the two countries are controlled. Table 3 shows that dialysis patients have an expected life 44.5 percent as long as the general population in Japan, while dialysis patients can expect to live only 15.3 percent as long as the general population in the US. Thus, although there is virtually no difference between the two societies in the life expectancies of the general populations for this middle-aged cohort, the Japanese dialysis patients can expect to live three times longer than the US dialysis patients.

Discussion

Previous research [1] has shown that survival of end-stage renal disease (ESRD) patients in the US is lower than corresponding estimates from Japan and the European Dialysis and Transplant Association (EDTA) countries after adjusting for age and diabetic status. The current study differs from the previous comparison to Japan in several ways. First, the prior study covered the earlier time period of 1982–87 rather than the more recent time period of 1988–89 in the current study. Second, the prior study focused on all modalities of care, i.e., all ESRD patients, while the current study focuses on dialysis patients only with adjustment for CAPD and hemodialysis. Third, the prior study included patients of all ages, while the current study focuses on middle-aged patients aged 45–64 years at onset of ESRD. Both studies focused on incident patient cohorts.

Middle-aged patients were selected for the current analysis for two reasons. First, transplantation is less common in this age group in the US than for younger patients. Second, in both Japan and the US it is believed that all patients experiencing renal failure in this age group are accepted for treatment, so the unmeasured selection factor can be minimized in these analyses as an explanation for the differences in survival.

The current results provide striking evidence that survival of dialysis patients in Japan is higher than in the US, whether measured on a comparative basis of dialysis patients in both countries or measured relative to the survival of the general population in both countries. The magnitude of the difference in survival, if taken at face value, is remarkable. These results suggest that if the Japanese experience can be generalized, then there may be substantial potential to improve the life expectancy of dialysis patients in the US, which is currently less than four years for all ESRD patients [4]. Prostate cancer patients in the US have a substantially longer life expectancy than dialysis patients in the US [4]. This statistic suggests that as an additional method of standardization it may be useful to compare dialysis patient survival in Japan with that for other maladies of the Japanese society.

Patterns in dialysis patient mortality in Japan suggest one of several possible explanations for the lower survival in the US: is there a potential for under-reporting of deaths in Japan during the time period of this study (1989)? Efforts to validate survival data have been made in both countries. A validation of US survival data for a national random sample of patients revealed a high rate of agreement between data from the Health Care Financing Administration and data obtained from the patients' medical records [14,15], while comparisons between national (JSDT) and regional area survival data in Japan and also in a recent report presented at the JSDT annual meeting [16] document the reliability of JSDT data. However, Japanese survival data for 1989 indicate a higher mortality rate during the second year compared to the first year following kidney failure. This pattern is different from the US and other registries, where first-year mortality tends to be higher than mortality in subsequent years. Both of these trends would be consistent with incomplete reporting of 1989 incident dialysis patient deaths to the JSDT during the first year if, for example, some patients who died early in their treatment history escaped reporting altogether, while patient deaths occurring during the second year following kidney failure were more likely to be documented. Supporting analyses, not presented, indicate that the survival of incident patients in Japan was longer for the 1989 cohort than for earlier cohorts (1983–88), although survival outcomes among earlier cohorts were still overall superior to US results. Future studies should attempt to confirm the relatively higher survival reported for the 1989 incident cohort in Japan compared to earlier incident cohorts.

Alternative explanations may exist for the relatively lower survival of dialysis patients in the US compared to Japan. The correction factor that was applied to US survival data (see Methods) to account for relatively higher mortality during the first 90 days following onset of ESRD lowered US survival relative to Japan. This correction factor has not been validated and may therefore either understate or overstate the true difference in mortality during the first 90 days compared to subsequent periods. However, this ratio is close to one (approximately 0.95) and is therefore unlikely to substantially overstate the observed difference in mortality. Dialysis patient mortality during the first 90 days in the US is a topic that merits further research.

Transplantation is very infrequent in Japan compared to the US [4]. It might be argued that the method of censoring transplanted patients in the US biases the US results to look comparatively worse, since transplantation selects the healthiest patients out of the dialysis population [3]. To test this hypothesis, the analysis was repeated without censoring at transplant, i.e., using an intent-to-treat specification model [17]. Under this specification, each patient remained in the same dialysis category until the end of the study, regardless of receipt of a transplanted organ. This alternative specification of an intent-to-treat model did not alter the basic conclusions of the current study, since for most subsets of patients US survival increased by less than one percentage point at one year and by approximately two percentage points at two years. Of the 16 disease/gender/age/modality groups in the current study, the increase in US survival that resulted from this change in specification was pronounced in only one case (i.e., more than one and three percentage points at one and two years, respectively).

Adequacy of dialysis in the US is an issue of continuing controversy [18], with many reports suggesting that the relatively higher mortality in the US can be attributed to inadequate dialysis. Possible explanations for differences in the quality of treatment include differences in the surface area of dialyzers, the duration of hemodialysis treatments, the practice of dialyzer reuse, and different financial systems that may result in different acceptance criteria. A recent study suggested that the length of hemodialysis treatments was shorter on average in the US than in Europe [19]. At a median of 9.8 hours per week (mean = 9.0 hours), this measure of treatment time also appears to be shorter than corresponding estimates in Japan. Future research should focus on factors such as these to determine whether more adequate dialysis treatments in Japan provide a major explanation for lower dialysis patient mortality reported for Japan compared to the US.

References

1. Held PJ, Brunner F, Odaka M, Garcia JR, Port FK, Gaylin DS. Five-year survival for end-stage renal disease patients in the United States, Europe, and Japan, 1982 to 1987. Am J Kidney Dis 1990; 15: 451–457.
2. Dialysis Mortality: Preventable or Inevitable? SUNY Health Science Center at Brooklyn, NY; April 26, 1993.
3. Gaylin DS, Held PJ, Port FK, Hunsicker LG, Wolfe RA, Kahan BD, Jones CA, Agodoa LYC. The impact of comorbid factors on access to renal transplantation. JAMA 1993; 269: 603–608.
4. United States Renal Data System. USRDS 1993 Annual Data Report. National Institutes of Health, National Institute of Diabetes and Digestive and Kidney Diseases, Bethesda, MD, March, 1993.
5. Japanese Society for Dialysis Therapy.
6. US Department of Health and Human Services, Health Care Financing Administration, Baltimore, MD; ESRD Program Medical Management and Information System, Computer Update, May 1992.
7. Kaplan EL, Meier P. Nonparametric estimation from incomplete observations. J Am Stat Assoc 53: 457–481.
8. Lawless, JF. Statistical Models and Methods for Lifetime Data, first edition. New York: John Wiley & Sons, 1982.
9. SAS Institute Inc. SAS User's Guide: Statistics, version 5 edition. Cary, NC: SAS Institute Inc., 1985.
10. United States Renal Data System. USRDS 1991 Annual Data Report. The National Institutes of Health, National Institute of Diabetes and Digestive and Kidney Diseases, Bethesda, MD, August 1991.
11. National Center for Health Statistics. Vital statistics of the United States, 1988, vol II, mortality, part A. Washington: Public Health Service, 1991.
12. Kokumin-eisei no doukou (Indexes of Public Health), vol 38, 1991.
13. US Bureau of the Census. Statistical abstract of the United States: 1991 (111th edition). Washington, DC, 1991.
14. United States Renal Data System. USRDS 1992 Annual Data Report. How good are the data? USRDS data validation special study. Am J Kidney Dis 1992; 20 (Suppl 2): 68–83.
15. United States Renal Data System. USRDS 1992 Annual Data Report. Completeness and reliability of USRDS data: comparisons with the Michigan Kidney Registry. Am J Kidney Dis 1992; 20 (Suppl 2): 84–88.
16. Report from Touseki-Ikai at JSDT 1992 annual meeting.
17. Nelson CB, Port FK, Wolfe RA, Guire KE. Comparison of CAPD and hemodialysis patient survival with evaluation of trends during the 1980s. J Am Soc Nephrol 1992; 3: 1147–1155.
18. Held PJ, Levin NW, Bovbjerg RR, Pauly MV, Diamond LH. Mortality and duration of hemodialysis treatment. JAMA 1991; 7: 871–875.
19. Held PJ, Blagg CR, Liska DW, Port FK, Hakim R, Levin NW. The dose of hemodialysis according to dialysis prescription in Europe and the United States. Kidney Int 1992; 42: S16–S21.

CHAPTER 3

Analysis of causes of death and of the direction of management to improve survival

Data from European Renal Association Registry (ERA–EDTA)

N.P. MALLICK, E.P. BRUNNER, E. JONES and N.H. SELWOOD

In recent years, European data has not been collected comprehensively and this has led to some difficulties in interpretation. The reason for this incompleteness is one of communication across thirty six countries and is being addressed. Numerically the data file is very large nevertheless and at the end of 1991 158,094 patients were recorded as alive on therapy. Internal evidence from the few large countries for which data is not complete suggests that the recorded data still represents about 85% of all patients on therapy in Europe.

The pattern of European data has been presented quite recently [1]. We have updated these analyses for this report.

Centre-based maintenance haemodialysis (MHD) remains the most frequent mode of renal replacement therapy (RRT) in Europe. Continuous ambulatory peritoneal dialysis (CAPD) is used now for a relatively stable proportion of European patients, being favoured particularly in the United Kingdom and Italy. Transplantation is pursued in all parts of Europe but is a proportionately more frequent mode of RRT in Scandinavia, Austria and the UK. A particular logistic – and moral – problem in Europe is the movement of patients maintained on dialysis in one country to another for transplantation, since this puts additional pressure on the generally limited availability of cadaver renal grafts in the host country. This adds too to the difficulties in ensuring that expert follow-up is maintained and complications recorded.

The death rate on RRT is clearly influenced by age (Fig. 1). While this is hardly surprising in that natural life span is shorter and the chance of coincidental non-renal disease (comorbidity) is greater as patients age, the full explanation for this phenomenon may not have been delineated, for age appears to be a risk factor independent of other influences (see Fig. 3).

Death rate is influenced by time on RRT. Figure 2 shows that for all ages, though at different percentage levels, on uninterrupted haemodialysis there is a higher mortality in the first year on treatment. Further analysis has suggested that cardiovascular causes are particularly important at this time.

E. A. Friedman (ed.), Death on Hemodialysis, 25–33.
© 1994 *Kluwer Academic Publishers.*

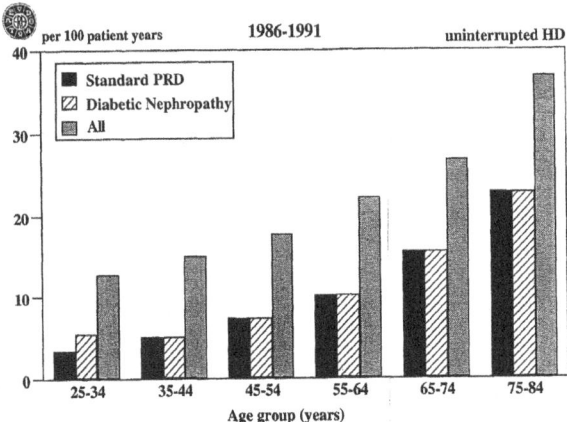

Fig. 1.   Mean annual mortality (per 100 patient years) during first five year period of uninterrupted haemodialysis for all patients starting renal replacement therapy during 1986 to 1991.

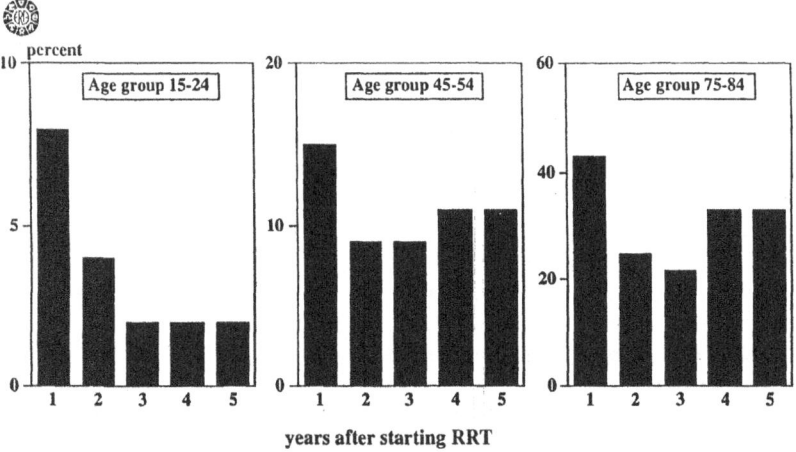

Fig. 2.   Annual mortality of patients on uninterrupted haemodialysis after start of renal replacement therapy in 1986.

Figure 3 demonstrates in the first few years on RRT there is an age related hierarchy for survival. For patients aged greater than 65, survival at five years is approximately one half that for patients aged less than 35. These are mean survivals and raise the question as to the care needed in selecting from these older patients those for whom therapy is likely to produce extended survival, together with a worthwhile quality of life.

The influence of particular diseases on mortality is of importance. The reported causes of end-stage renal failure (ESRF) in different European coun-

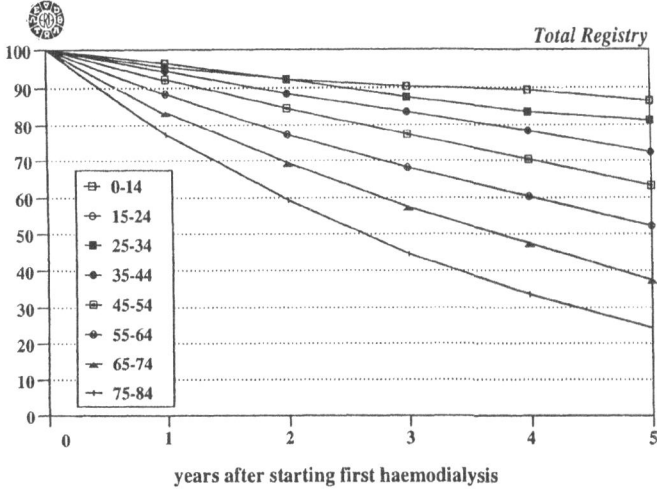

Fig. 3.   Survival on haemodialysis: all patients beginning renal replacement therapy during 1986 to 1991.

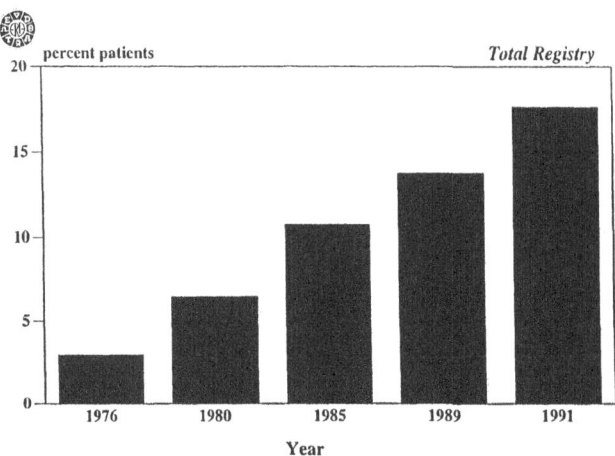

Fig. 4.   All patients with diabetic end-stage renal failure accepted for renal replacement therapy in the year specified.

tries differs markedly for some diseases Table 1 yet is relatively stable for such conditions as polycystic disease. The incidence of diabetes, and so of diabetic nephropathy, is higher in some Scandinavian countries, especially Finland, and affects the pattern of care required in managing ESRF. At the end of 1991 diabetes mellitus accounted for 8.1% of the stock of patients on RRT in Europe and 14.4% of patients reported to us as commencing RRT between 1.1.91 and 31.12.91 (Fig. 4).

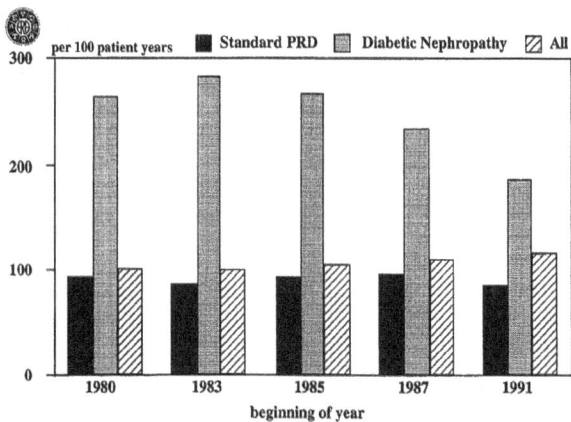

Fig. 5. Annual death rate (per 100 patient years) of all patients on haemodialysis according to primary renal disease.

Table 1. Differences in the perceived cause of end-stage renal failure in different countries.

	Primary Renal Disease Percent patients starting RRT in 1990				
	Glomerulonephritis	Pyelonephritis	Cystic	Vascular	Diabetes
Spain	19	14	10	12	13
Poland	52	15	8	3	6
Bulgaria	23	45	11	1	10
Finland	19	9	9	8	25

The death rate of diabetic patients on RRT is higher in any age cohort than the rate for patients with any other form of renal disease and this is multifactorial. The data in Fig. 5 suggests that, over the last few years, the management of diabetic patients on RRT has improved, for the annual mortality appears to be falling despite there being more and older patients on treatment.

The diabetic patient poses a complex problem. The aims of the St. Vincent's Declaration include a reduction by approximately 50% in the incidence of diabetic nephropathy, but this could only be achieved if there was vigorous management of the insulin dependent diabetic from the earliest detection of disease and the detection of covert non-insulin dependent diabetes mellitus in population related detection studies.

To prevent the progression of diabetic nephropathy, a team approach is needed in which the nephrologist and diabetic physician are partners. We in Europe are actively seeking to develop such teams and to follow prospectively in their work. This will enable us to develop clear guidelines for the expert

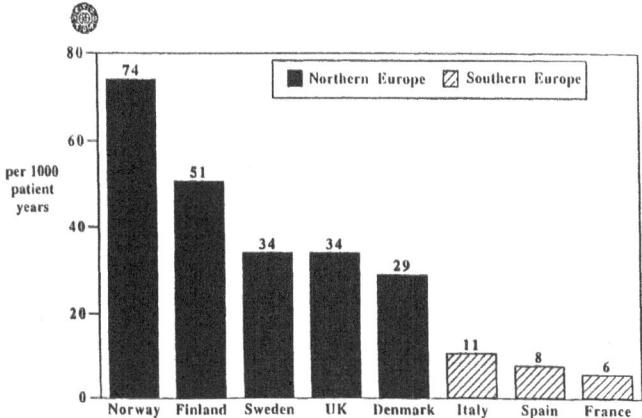

Fig. 6. Myocardial ischaemia/infarction annual death rates in males aged 35–64 years, all primary renal diseases, commencing renal replacement therapy during 1985 to 1990.

management of diabetic nephropathy in its earlier phases and this should improve the prognosis for the patient who does develop ESRF.

A further issue needing clarification is the clear definition of insulin and non-insulin dependent diabetes mellitus in the patient with renal impairment. This can be difficult if patients are seen only when renal failure is advised since insulin may then be required in any case. We in Europe hope to contribute to a more precise definition of the form of diabetes a given patient has since this will assess in determining the patterns of diabetes across Europe and in defining the problems which face patients with different forms of the disease.

It need hardly be stated that such an interventionist approach in the earlier phases of diabetes can only improve the survival and reduce the morbidity of the diabetic patient on RRT.

A concern to us has been the level of mortality and of morbidity from cardiovascular disease in ESRF. It is well documented that this is a problem in ESRF of any cause but particularly so in those with diabetes mellitus. The reported mortality rate of myocardial infarction is strikingly different across Europe, with a low rate in the Mediterranean and high rate in some of the more Northern European countries (Fig. 6). These differences await explanation. The increment due to ESRF is calculated to be about the same (some twenty times) both in Italy and the UK in males and females in the diabetic or non-diabetic subject. All comparisons are with the indigenous population but without renal failure. If there is ischaemic heart disease in the pre-end stage phase of renal impairment, the likelihood of this being a major factor in mortality and morbidity while on RRT is clearly increased [2,3]. Indeed, the absence of known risk factors for ischaemic heart disease in the pre-ESRF patient is good evidence that ischaemic heart disease will not be a problem after RRT has been initiated [2].

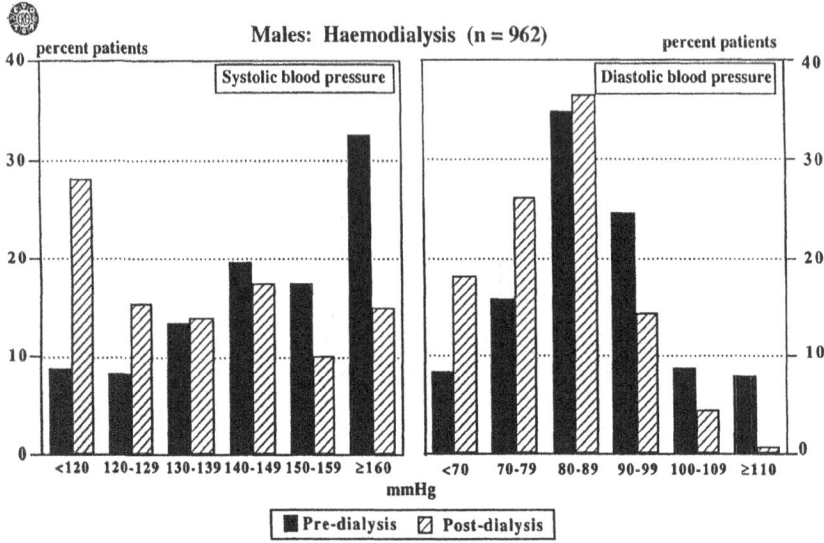

Fig. 7.   Distribution of most recent pre-dialysis and post-dialysis blood pressure in males on haemodialysis. Before dialysis 30% of patients had a systolic blood pressure below 140 mmHg, compared to 58% after dialysis.

This points to the need for nephrologists increasingly to ensure that patients with renal impairment are seen early in their course since morbidity on RRT then can be anticipated and minimized by good preventative measures or surgical intervention before RRT commences.

Hypertension is a recognised factor in cardiovascular disease. It is disturbing to see that blood pressure control is not always well maintained on haemodialysis (Fig. 7). There is need both to ensure adequate fluid removal – and discourage inappropriate fluid intake – and only when this has been achieved to introduce hypotensive agents as necessary. Again, we in Europe are developing a cohort base study to assess this and other cardiovascular risk factors in the medium to long-term outlook for our patients on RRT.

Transplantation has a major influence on the statistical analysis on the outcome of RRT. It is arguable that the most useful outcome parameter is the 'all-comers' one in which the 1, 5, 10 and 15 year prognosis for a patient joining an RRT program is calculated taking account of age at commencement of therapy but leaving the change of therapeutic mode within RRT to the educated (and of course changing) choice of patient and doctor together. On this basis, as Fig. 8 shows, patients and their relatives do have a reasonable chance of calculating the "average" risk and this can be refined in discussion with the physician to account for age, for the cause of renal disease (for example, diabetes mellitus) and for co-morbidity. However, if patients who have undergone transplantation are excluded, then the survivals on dialysis

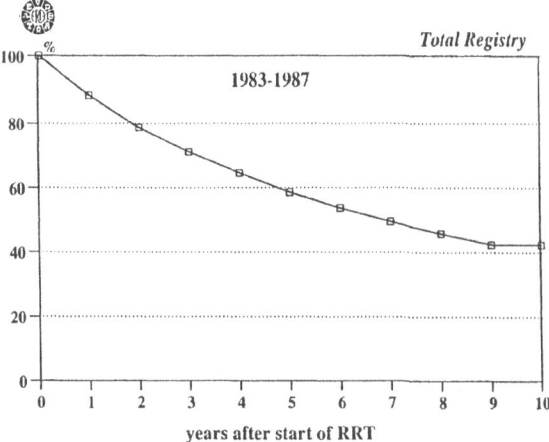

Fig. 8. Survival of patients commencing renal replacement therapy in 1983 to 1987 irrespective of changes in mode of therapy, (to the registry).

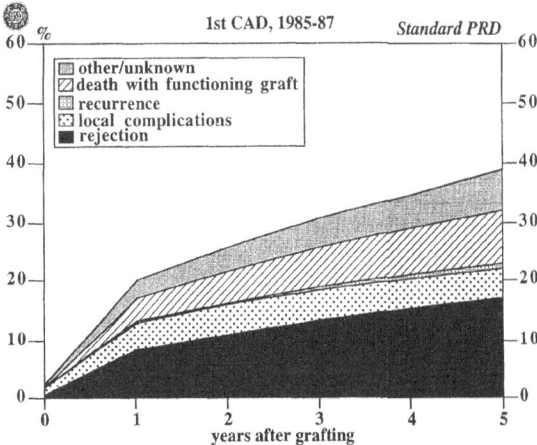

Fig. 9. Actuarial 1st cadaveric graft loss, standard PRD, 1985–1987.

alone may be influenced negatively by the selection out of the fittest patients for transplantation. International comparisons must account for this factor.

Figures 9 and 10 give a visual representation of the way in which underlying disease and co-morbidity influence survival with a successful graft, while Figs. 11 and 12 underline the place of cardiovascular disease especially in post graft mortality. These illustrations reinforce the point discussed earlier in this paper on the need for careful pre-end stage management in assessing and dealing with cardiovascular risk factor and of the careful assessment of these factors while on dialysis. Together these measures could prolong the

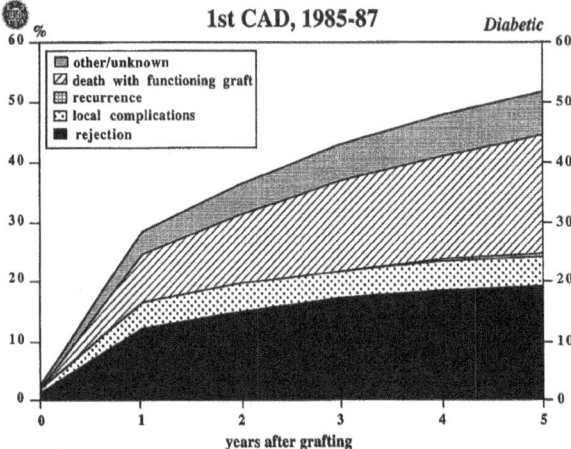

Fig. 10.   Actuarial 1st cadeveric graft loss, diabetic nephropathy, 1985–1987. For patients with diabetic nephropathy, the major cause of graft failure at five years was death with a functioning graft.

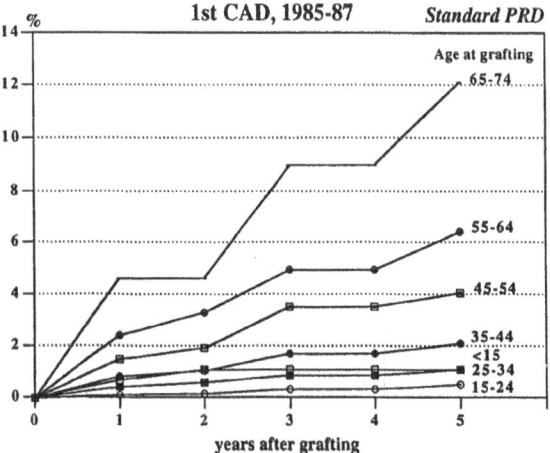

Fig. 11.   Actuarial death rate with functioning 1st cadaveric graft due to cardiovascular causes, standard PRD, from 1985–1987.

life of many grafts which are otherwise lost because patients have died of cardiovascular death.

Overall, survival on renal replacement therapy has been one of the success stories of the past few decades in medicine. The data presented here do not address in detail some of the underlying risks for survival. In particular we have not elaborated on the need to maintain good nutritional status and to tailor dialysis to ensure that the uraemic environment is reduced as much as

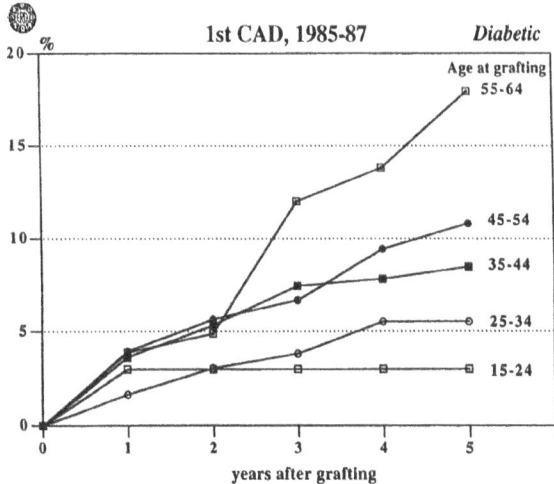

Fig. 12.   Actuarial death rate with functioning 1st cadaveric graft due to cardiovascular causes, diabetic nephropathy, from 1985–1987.

possible – and to introduce medical intervention where necessary with drugs to maintain clinical and metabolic status at an optimal level throughout. Studies in Europe are underway to assess these points more precisely, as they are in other parts of the world, and one can look for even better survival, with even better quality of life for our patients in the years to come.

References

1. Brunner FP, Selwood NH. Profile of patients on RRT in Europe and death rates due to major causes of death groups. Kidney Int 1992; 42 (Suppl 38): S4–S15.
2. Brown JH, Hunt LP, Vites NP *et al*. Comparative morbidity from cardiovascular disease in patients with chronic renal failure. (submitted).
3. Koch M, Thomas B, Tschope W *et al*. Survival and predictors of death in dialysed diabetic patients. (submitted).

CHAPTER 4

Treacherous fantasy:
The unfulfilled promise of Kt/V

We do not use nor do we need formulas

HANS J. GURLAND and SALIM K. MUJAIS

The position that we propose in this essay is that the various formulas developed for urea kinetic modeling, and the reliance thereon, are an impediment rather than a help in the determination of a proper dialysis prescription. Such a position, we must herein rapidly admit, should not be considered as immutable or universal for such would be contrary to critical thinking. In medical issues, one must abandon the framework of strict truth and untruth and adopt what has been whimsically called "Fuzzy truth" [1]. The simile for this is that if one considers truth as having a value of 1, and untruth as having a value of zero, then "fuzzy truth" can have a value between 0.1 and 0.9, hence one abandons the binary system for the fractional system. Along these lines one can rephrase the title to state that we almost never use formulas (a fuzzy truth value of 0.7!) and they are almost never useful (a fuzzy truth value of 0.65!).

The evaluation of the usefulness of urea kinetic formulas should take into account the following caveat:

1. The validation of the theoretical basis of these formulas;
2. Distinction between use for research and use as a clinical prescription tool;
3. The role of these formulas in the complex setting of therapeutic decisions and the variety of factors, medical and otherwise that govern dialysis prescription. Under this heading one must examine such factors as the requirements of reimbursing agencies and the like.

Kt/V: theoretical and practical limitations

Before considering the various formulas and the theoretical arguments presented for their validity, it is important to point out that urea kinetic formulas seem to represent an 'American' phenomenon (Fig. 1). A review of the studies published between 1980 and 1992 and listed in Medline dealing with the theoretical basis of urea kinetics reveals a predominance of US studies in this field. Further, it should be pointed out that some of the studies from certain European countries represent the repeated efforts of a single center

E. A. Friedman (ed.), Death on Hemodialysis, 35–43.
© 1994 *Kluwer Academic Publishers.*

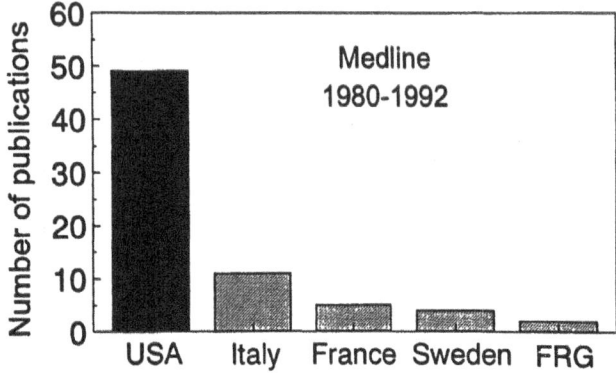

Fig. 1.   Number of publications listed in Medline appearing between 1980 and 1992 dealing with the subject of urea kinetic modeling in uremia and the value of Kt/V, categorized by country of origin.

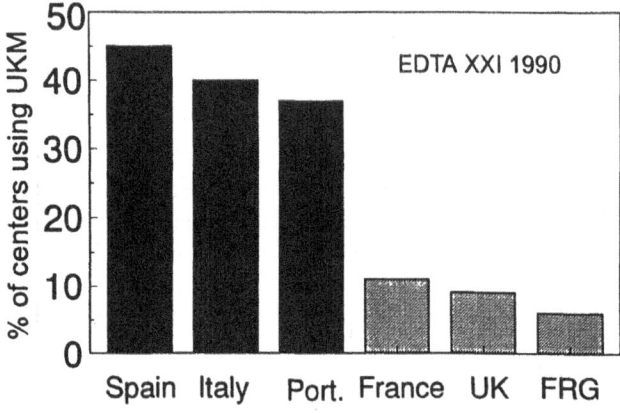

Fig. 2.   Use of urea kinetic modeling in dialysis centers in Europe in 1990 [2]. The percentages refer to centers that use urea kinetic modeling on most of their patients. The preferred modality is Kt/V.

and frequently a single investigator (for example Italy and Sweden), whereas the studies from the US reflect a rather widespread interest in the topic.

Within Europe, there seems to be a heterogeneity in the frequency of clinical use of urea kinetic modeling (Fig. 2). While southern European countries have a medium level of usage, the practice is exceedingly rare in northern Europe [2]. The pattern in northern Europe parallels the paucity of academic interest in the field. One is tempted to speculate on the reasons for the disparity between northern and southern Europe, and it is not unlikely that economic factors may play a role. While generally considered to be very common, the exact frequency of utilization of urea kinetic modeling in the

Table 1. Formulas for Kt/V calculation

Formula	Author
Kt/V = ln(Upre/Upost)	(Gotch 85)
Kt/V = 0.04 PRU–1.2	(Jindal 87)
Kt/V = (Upre–Upost)/Umid	(Barth 88)
Kt/V = -ln(R–0.008t–UF/W)	(Daugirdas 89)
Kt/V = =ln(R–0.03–UF/W)	(Manahan 89)
Kt/V = 0.026 PRU–0.46	(Daugirdas 90)
Kt/V = 0.023 PRU–0.284	(Basile 90)
Kt/V = 0.062 PRU–2.97	(Kerr 93)

Upre and Upost refer to blood urea concentration
values before and after dialysis.
Umid refers to midpoint blood urea concentration.
PRU is the percent reduction in urea calculated as
PRU = (Upre–Upost) * 100/Upre. t refers to time
on dialysis, W to body weight, UF to ultrafiltration
volume, and R to ratio Upost/Upre.

US is not known, but if the trend towards regulatory control by the Health
Care Financing Administration (HCFA) is any indication, the practice may
soon become universal.

The number of formulas recommended for evaluation of urea kinetics
continues to rise (Table 1) [3–10]. While several of these are variants of each
other, the continuing search for the easiest and most accurate formula reflects,
in our opinion, an underlying uneasiness about these formulas in general, or
a need to maximize their use by minimizing the burden of calculation. The
trend has been to suggest simpler and simpler formulas. But to quote Friedrich
Nietzsche, "Simplification is falsification".

The choice of a particular formula, which is frequently random in clinical
practice or possibly governed by non-scientific reasons, such as the availability of a certain computer software, or a personal bias towards a certain author,
may engender problems. Kerr *et al.* [10] have illustrated the variability in
Kt/V estimation by comparing the results obtained by standard urea kinetic
modeling and 3 formulas. The results obtained in the same patients by application of different formulas vary from 1.3 to 1.7 (Fig. 3, open bars)! Even for
a single formula, the value of Kt/V depends on so many minor factors that
serious errors are likely to occur more frequently than is generally recognized.
A common limitation is the phenomenon of urea rebound that occurs after the
end of dialysis. Initial reports had suggested that it is in the order of 10% and
therefore can be safely ignored without untoward consequences [11]. Recent
studies, however, suggest that – especially in fast dialysis – it can be as high
as 25% [10]. The consequence of rebound on Kt/V calculation is illustrated in
Fig. 3. Utilization of urea values obtained immediately at the end of dialysis
leads consistently to overestimation of Kt/V irrespective of the formula used
compared to urea values obtained 30 minutes after the termination of dialysis
and after equilibration [10]. In the practical world, immediate urea values

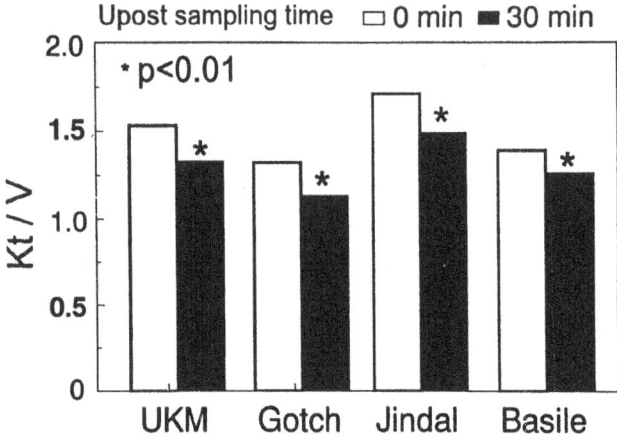

Fig. 3.   Variability in Kt/V estimation and effect of urea rebound [10]. Open bars represent Kt/V calculated on the same patient population with standard urea kinetic modeling (UKM) or by 3 proposed formulas using end of dialysis blood urea concentration (Upost sampling time 0 min,). Filled bars reflect corresponding values obtained using blood urea concentration measured 30 min after the termination of dialysis (Upost sampling time 30 min).

Table 2. Pitfalls in urea kinetic determinations

Urea rebound
Single pool model of urea kinetics
Errors in time registration
Errors in blood flow measurements
Recirculation
Estimates of body water
Residual renal function
Use of manufacturer clearances
Intradialytic catabolism

Upre and Upost refer to blood urea concentration values before and after dialysis.
Umid refers to midpoint blood urea concentration.
PRU is the percent reduction in urea calculated as PRU = (Upre–Upost) * 100/Upre. t refers to time on dialysis, W to body weight, UF to ultrafiltration volume, and R to ratio Upost/Upre.

are obtained as keeping dialysis patients for an additional 30 minutes with a vascular access is rarely met with benign acceptance!

Additional pitfalls in urea kinetic determinations are listed in Table 2. While most intradialytic and interdialytic evaluations suggest that a two pool model is more appropriate for urea [12], dialysis experts continue to use a single pool model [13], likely because of the added mathematical complexity of multiple pool models, and a complex formula is rarely used by busy clinicians! Time on dialysis is frequently and almost consistently overestimated. Blood flow indicators on dialysis machines are not very accurate and flow is not constant during a dialysis session. Attention to recirculation is rare except in very few patients in whom clinical suspicion of recirculation warrants a formal evaluation.

The volume of distribution of urea, assumed to be total body water, is subject to many variables. The effects of age and gender in normal individuals have been known since the fifties [14], but are frequently ignored. But even the validity of the determinations in normal individuals to assessment of body water in uremic subjects is questionable. Further, body water is constantly varying in dialyzed patients.

Manufacturer provided clearances are frequently measured under optimal in vitro conditions. Real *in vivo* values during dialysis are thought to be 20% lower, and an error of equal magnitude is introduced in urea kinetic modeling if the *in vitro* values are used. Residual renal function and intradialytic catabolism are additional variables that need to be accounted for in any careful determination of urea kinetics.

Kt/V: research vs, clinical prescription tool

An intriguing limitation of the use of Kt/V lies in the analysis and interpretation of this tool in research studies. A prototype of this is the analysis of the National Cooperative Dialysis Study (NCDS) [3,15]. Before we discuss the variable analysis of this landmark study, it is important to stress that the distinction between a research tool used under controlled conditions and for defined purposes of comparative study or tracking of effect within defined limits, and a clinical decision tool used in a complex setting with many intangible variables, should always be kept in mind. The conditions under which a tool is valid in a research setting may not obtain in the clinical sphere. Further, the limited defined objectives assigned to a tool in the research setting, cannot be transposed easily to clinical goals of therapy.

Two different experts [3,15], analyzing the same data have arrived at two different conclusions (Fig. 4). The difference is not negligible. If you accept that Kt/V is a discontinuous function [3] with no further benefit above a certain level, then therapy is limited to achievement of the presumed critical level. If you believe it is a continuous function [15], then the clinical decision is to continue to increase the value of Kt/V for a particular patient as further benefit is thereby accrued.

Role of UKM formulas in therapeutic decisions

The crucial point of the controversy about these formulas is clearly whether they should guide our therapeutic decisions. The lack of use of urea kinetic modeling formulas in northern Europe has not had a negative impact on patient morbidity survival, and their frequent use in the US has not provided a safety net for US patients.

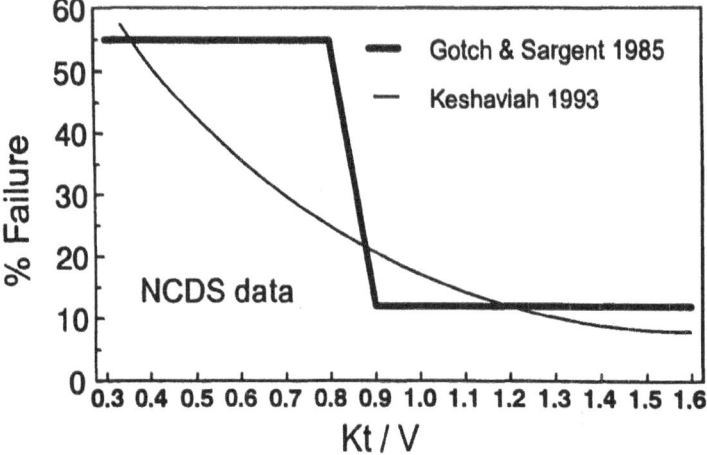

Fig. 4. Analysis of Kt/V from the NCDS study revealing either a discontinuous function [3] or a continuous function [15].

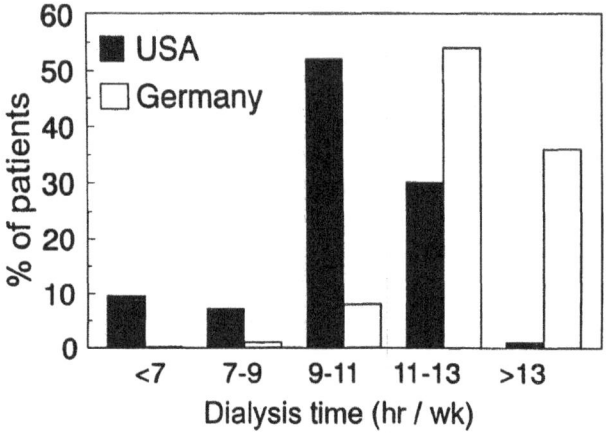

Fig. 5. Total weekly dialysis time in the United States and Germany [2,16,17]. The percentage of the total patients in each time group is represented by the bars.

It is readily clear to all practiced physicians that the labeling of our field as an 'Art and a Science' is not accidental. Our medical forefathers must have recognized the non-scientific factors that become entangled in our practice, and quite creatively labeled them as 'the Art of Medicine', basically to camouflage uncertainty, or erratic behavior, under a mantle of lofty colors. The answer to the above stated questions must lie in an examination of what really determines the clinical practice of dialysis.

It is instructive to reflect on the differences in dialysis prescription between the users of urea kinetic modeling (US) and the non-users (Europe and specif-

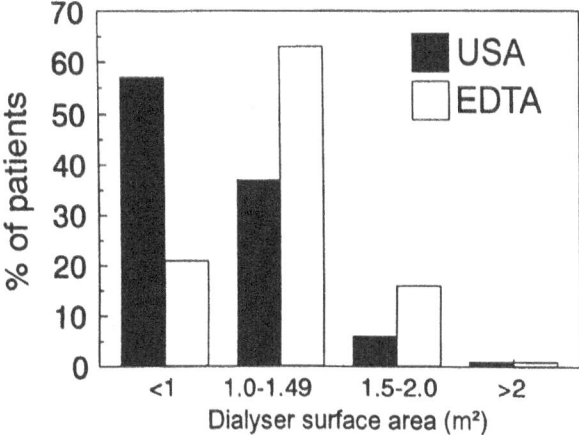

Fig. 6.   Dialyser surface area in the United States and Europe [2,16,17]. The percentage of the total patients in each range of dialyser surface area is represented by the bars.

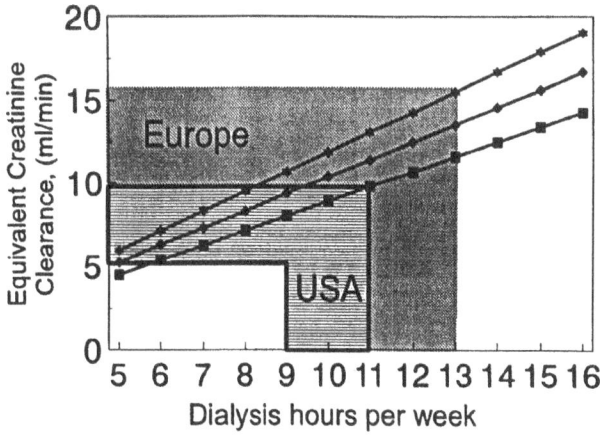

Fig. 7.   Equivalent creatinine clearance provided by the total dialytic therapy in the US and Europe. This value is calculated by dividing total weekly creatinine clearance provided by the dialyser by the total number of minutes per week and is broadly equivalent to endogenous residual renal function of the patient. Distinct areas of operations can be delineated for US and Europe based on dialysis time and the range of used dialyser surface area and creatinine clearance. Three representative values for dialyser creatinine clearances are depicted in the line plots: stars for dialyser creatinine clearance of 200 ml/min, diamonds for dialyser creatinine clearance of 175 ml/min., and squares for dialyser creatinine clearance of 150 ml/min.

ically Germany). The distribution of cumulative weekly time on dialysis for German patients (Fig. 5) is clearly shifted to the right (longer time) compared to US subjects, with the majority of patients in Germany dialyzing for more than 11 hours, whereas the majority of patients in the US dialyze for less than 11 hours [2,16,17]. The effect of dialysis time is magnified by the observation that dialysers of larger surface area are also used in Europe compared to the US (Fig. 6) [2,16,17]. The combined effect of these two parameters is that German nephrologists who do not use urea kinetic modeling prescribe more dialysis for their patients than US nephrologists who frequently use these formulas! This is illustrated by the concept of the equivalent creatinine clearance that represents the equivalent endogenous renal function provided by total weekly hemodialysis when dialysis time and dialyser creatinine clearance are known (Fig. 7). Values for European patients aggregate in an area distinct from that of US patients.

It is becoming increasingly clear that financial factors play a more important role than many would like to admit, and erosion of financial support does threaten the quality of delivery of care [18,19]. The financial constraints imposed on US nephrologists are significantly greater than other post-industrial societies [18,19], and the impact of these constraints on the outcome of dialysis is a subject of ongoing debate [19] with very clear political overtones!

The influence of limited resources is compounded by the economic behavior of the health care providers. The majority of ESRD facilities in the US are run for profit and the average number of patients per for profit facility is greater than the corresponding number in nonprofit facilities [19]. The opposite of that is true for Germany. Furthermore, a greater proportion of for profit facilities with a lower financial support is a prescription for trouble. Witness the high frequency of reuse in for profit facilities compared to nonprofit and hospital based units [19]. While the issue of reuse will be dealt with by other contributors to this volume, it may be sobering to compare reuse policies between different nations. The US is in that aspect comparable to the poorest East European countries (Poland and Bulgaria) and stands in contrast to West European nations [2,19].

In conclusion, the danger of reliance on urea kinetic modeling and the various simplified formulas is that it may provide a false sense of safety and lull the physicians into believing that adequate care is being delivered. While urea kinetic modeling may be a useful adjunct under very limited conditions, its danger in practice is greater than its benefit. The danger is that regulatory agencies may utilize this index as a criterion for continued financial support and as a quality assurance tool, and then, the hand that holds the economic rope would be tightening the noose on proper ESRD therapy.

Acknowledgment

The authors would like to thank the following individuals for helpful comments and provision of valuable data for the preparation of this review: A. Peter Lundin, MD, State University of New York, New York, USA; Rudolf Nardei, Kuratorium fur Dialyse und Nieren Transplantation, Neu Isenburg, FRG; Hiroshi Tanaka, MD, Ph.D., Ohno Memorial Hospital, Osaka, Japan; Richard Ward Ph.D., University of Louisville, Louisville, Kentucky, USA.

References

1. Stewart I. Mathematical recreations: a partly true story. Scientific American 1993; 268(2): 110–112.
2. Geerlings W, Tufveson G, Brunner FP, Ehrich JHH, Fassbinder W, Landais P, Mallick N, Margreiter R, Raine AEG, Rizzoni G, Selwood N. Combined report on regular dialysis and transplantation in Europe, XXI, 1990.
3. Gotch F, Sargent J. A mechanistic analysis of the National Cooperative Dialysis Study. Kidney Int 1985; 28: 526–534.
4. Jindal KK, Manuel A, Goldstein MB. Percent reduction in blood urea concentration during hemodialysis: a simple and accurate method to estimate Kt/V. Trans Am Soc Art Intern Organs 1987; 33; 286–288.
5. Barth RH. Direct calculation of Kt/V. A simplified approach to monitoring of hemodialysis. Nephron 1988; 50: 191–195.
6. Daugirdas JT. Bedside formulas for Kt/V. A kinder, gentler approach to urea kinetic modeling. ASAIO Trans 1989; 35: 336–338.
7. Manahan FJ, Ramanujam L, Ajam M, Ing TD, Ghandi VC, Daugirdas JT. Post to predialysis plasma urea nitrogen ratio, ultrafiltration and weight to estimate Kt/V ASAIO Trans 1989; 35: 511–512.
8. Daugirdas JT. Rapid methods of estimating Kt/V: three formulas compared. ASAIO Trans 1990; 36: M362–M364.
9. Basile C, Casino F, Lopez T. Percent reduction in blood urea concentration during hemodialysis estimates Kt/V in a simple and accurate way. Am J Kidney Dis 1990; 15: 40–45.
10. Kerr PG, Argiles A, Canaud B, Flavier JL, Mion CM. Accuracy of Kt/V estimations in high flux haemodiafiltration using percent reduction of urea: incorporation of urea rebound. Nephrol Dial Transplant 1993; 8: 149–153.
11. Pedrini LA, Zereik S, Ramsey S. Causes, kinetics and clinical implications of post hemodialysis urea rebound. Kidney Int 1988; 34: 817–824.
12. Vanholder RC, Ringoir S. Adequacy of dialysis: a critical analysis. Kidney Int 1992; 42: 540–558.
13. Hakim R. Assessing the adequacy of dialysis. Kidney Int 1990; 37: 822–832.
14. Edelman IS, Haley HB, Schloerb PR, Sheldon DB, Friihansen BJ, Stoll G, Moore FD. Further observations on total body water. I. Normal values throughout life span. Surg Gynecol Obstetr 1952; 95: 1–12.
15. Keshaviah P. Urea kinetic and middle molecule approaches to assessing the adequacy of hemodialysis and CAPD. Kidney Int 1993; 43 (Suppl 40): S28–S38.
16. US Renal Data System, (USRDS) Annual Data Report. Characteristics of dialysis prescriptions in the US 1986–1987. Am J Kidney Dis 1992; 20: 39–47.
17. Held PJ, Levin NW, Bovbjerg RR, Pauly M, Diamond LH. Mortality and duration of hemodialysis treatment. JAMA 1991; 265: 871–875.
18. Nissenson AR, Prichard SS, Cheng IKP, Gokal R, Kubota M, Maiorca R, Riella MC, Rottembourg J, Stewart J. Non-medical factors that impact ESRD modality selection. Kidney Int 1993; 43 (Suppl 40): S120–S127.
19. Iglehart JK. The End Stage Renal Disease program. New Engl J Med 1993; 328: 366–371.

CHAPTER 5

ESRD registry statistics on dialysis mortality in Japan

FUMIAKI MARUMO, KENJI MAEDA and SHOZO KOSHIKAWA

Introduction

Survival of patients on dialysis therapy for end-stage renal disease (ESRD) has been a main concern of nephrologists and physicians [1–9]. The steady increase in continuous ambulatory peritoneal dialysis (CAPD) patients made it possible to compare outcomes of CAPD patients and hemodialysis patients. The United States Renal Data System (USRDS), established in 1988, has begun to supply excellent-quality statistics on dialysis therapy. Analysis of these data revealed many determinants in morbidity and mortality of dialysis patients: dialyzer reuse, duration of dialysis, quality of dialyzer membranes, causes of ESRD, availability of transplantation, and the age distribution of background population.

Simple comparisons of gross mortalities from the USRDS, European Dialysis Transplantation Association (EDTA), the Canadian Survey, and Japanese Society for Dialysis Therapy (JSDT) revealed that mortality of US ESRD patients is strikingly different compared with other countries, although survey methods used differed in these surveys.

The purpose of this report is to characterize the JSDT Annual Survey of Dialysis Patients and to analyze the mortality of Japanese ESRD patients on dialysis therapy.

Methods

Data of this analysis were mainly from Annual Reports of the Survey Committee of the JSDT from 1983–1991 [10–12]. The JSDT Survey Committee annually sent a questionnaire regarding chronic dialysis therapy to all facilities that conducted dialysis therapy based on the JSDT membership, dialysate customer lists, and a list of facilities to whom patients were transferred. Questionnaire items were characterization of the facility, patient numbers, sex, age, original diseases, start date of dialysis therapy, modality, outcome, and some

45

E. A. Friedman (ed.), Death on Hemodialysis, 45–54.
© 1994 *Kluwer Academic Publishers.*

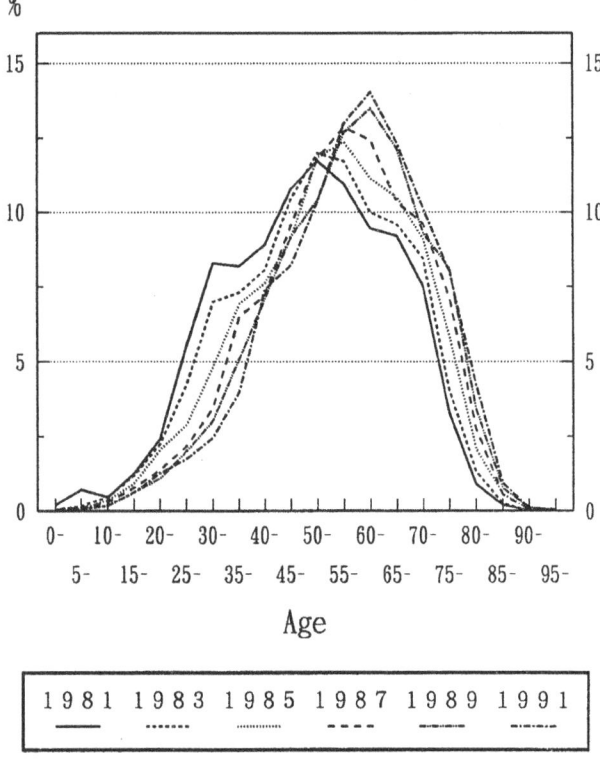

Fig. 1.   Incidence of chronic dialysis patients by age in Japan from 1983 to 1991.

special-theme items. Recovery of questionnaires and quality of the responses were confirmed by regional committee members, which were composed of more than fifty nephrologists. We also started personal follow-ups of patients identified by Kanji characters of patients' name and birthday beginning in 1983. Longitudinal data of 131,585 ESRD patients on dialysis therapy were accumulated as records on a magnetic tape that will be kept available for future analysis.

Results

Fundamental description

The recovery of questionnaires ranged from 95% to 99.3%. A total of 20,877 patients started dialysis therapy and 9,722 patients died in 1991. The number of ESRD patients was 116,303 on December 31, 1991, reaching 937.6 patients per million of the Japanese population. Dialysis therapy started at age 58.15 ± 14.58 year (mean ± S.D.) in 1991 which was 6.23 years later than that in 1983 (51.92 ± 15.54 years) (Fig. 1) [13]. Age distribution

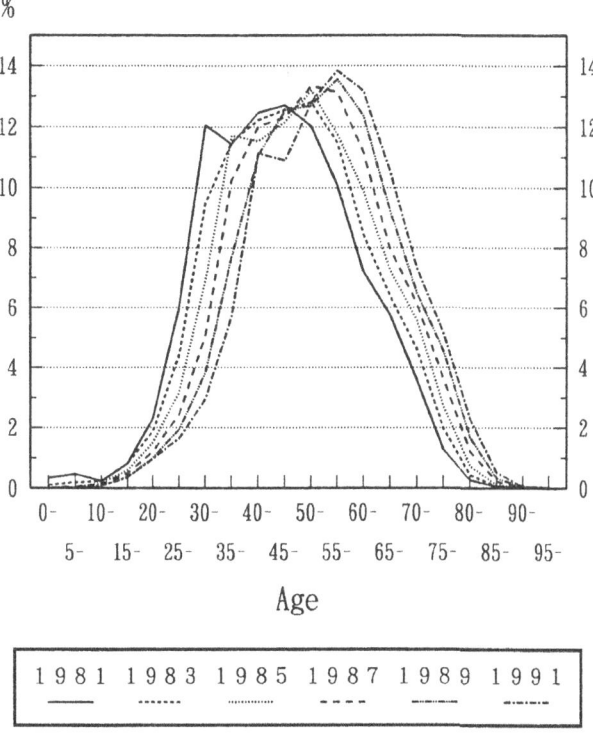

%

Fig. 2.   Living dialysis patients on December 31, by age in Japan from 1983 to 1991.

of patients on dialysis therapy shifted to the right with the average age of 48.25 ± 13.84 in 1983 rising to 55.29 ± 13.54 years in 1991 (Fig. 2). The original diseases that resulted in ESRD have changed. 58.3 per cent of ESRD patients' diseases was caused by chronic glomerulonephritis in 1983. In 1991, chronic glomerulonephritis only accounted for 44.1% of ESRD diseases, and 27.8% of new ESRD patients' diseases was caused by diabetes mellitus (DM).

Financial/reimbursement

Seventy to 100% of the cost of all medical fees was paid by public health insurance in Japan. Typical reimbursements for hemodialysis therapy and CAPD were respectively 454,000 yen/month/patient (3,996 dollars/month/patient) and 468,000 yen/month/patient (4,120 dollars/month/patient). The rest of the cost which was not covered by public insurance, was subsidized by the government from the start of dialysis therapy, resulting in virtually no private charge. Other social and economical supports, like transportation to hospitals and home-care service, were supplied as national and regional service.

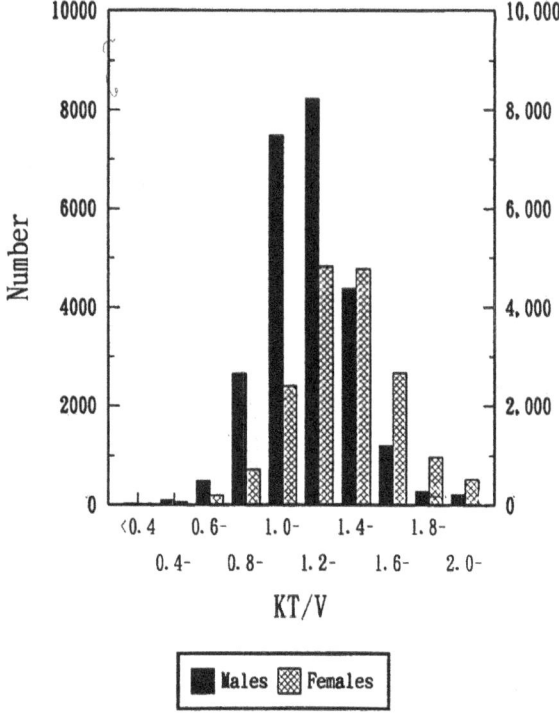

Fig. 3.   Distribution of Kt/V by age and gender in Japan in ESRD patients with nominal residual urine that were treated by hemodialysis three times a week.

ESRD modality and dose of therapy

ESRD patients were treated using daytime hospital hemodialysis (83, 373 patients; 71.7%), nighttime hospital hemodialysis (27, 397 patients; 23.6%), home hemodialysis (37 patients, <0.1%), CAPD (5; 427 patients; 4.7%) and IPD (64 patients; 0.1%). Sixty-five per cent of chronic dialysis patients were treated by private (profit) facilities. The total maximum capacity of all hemodialysis facilities was 143,760 hemodialysis patients.

The dose of hemodialysis therapy was examined with a single pool urea kinetic modeling in dialysis patients with nominally no urine production who were treated three times a week [14]. Duration of each hemodialysis was 4.30 $\pm$ 0.57 hours ($n = 42, 116$ patients), with post-dialysis patients body weight of 51.43 $\pm$ 9.28 kg. Pre-dialysis concentrations of blood urea nitrogen were 79.68 $\pm$ 17.75 mg/dl ($n = 42, 116$). Kt/V values were 1.25 $\pm$ 0.26 ($n = 25, 011$) in males and 1.42 $\pm$ 0.31 in females ($n = 17, 105$) (Fig. 3). Those were not different between age groups except a slight decrease in the over–75 age group. Over 98% of hemodialysis patients, who were treated three times a week, satisfied the standard from the NCDS guideline (Kt/V $>= 0.8$) [15].

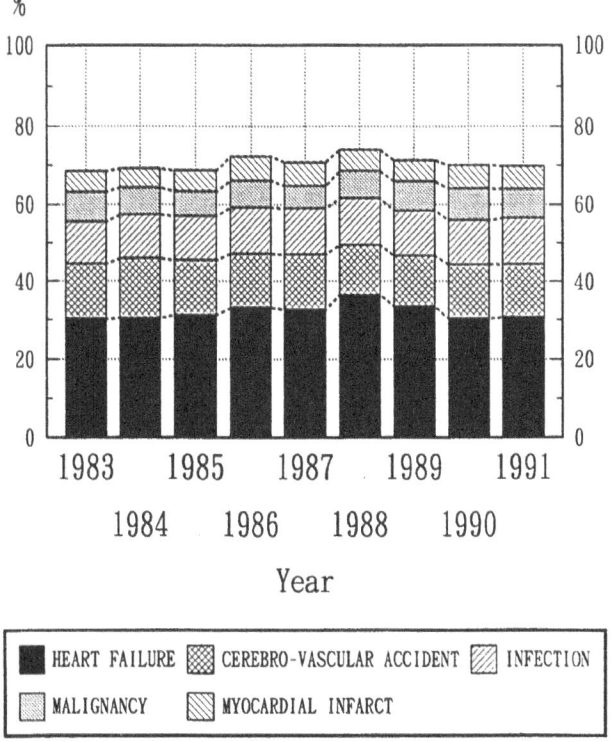

Fig. 4.   Changes in main causes of death for dialysis patients in Japan 1983–1991.

Protein catabolic rates of these patients were 1.01 ± 0.20 g/kg/day, and over 88% satisfied the guideline from the NCDS (PCR> = 0.8 kg/day)(16). No significant differences of PCR were observed in gender, age, original diseases, or age at start of hemodialysis.

Cause of death

Causes of death in 1991 were reported in 9,407 of 9,722 patients. They were heart failure (30.7%), cerebrovascular accidents (13.7%), infection (12.1%), malignancy (7.6%), uremia (6.5%), myocardial infarction (5.8%) and bleeding (3.1%) (Fig. 5).

To confirm the reliability of these reports, causes of death in 2,851 patients, who were autopsied in 1991, were analyzed. The causes were congestive heart failure (26.1%), cerebrovascular accident (18.7%), malignancy (13.3%), pneumonia (8.7%), sepsis (7.8%), and myocardial infarction/cardiomyopathy (7.0%).

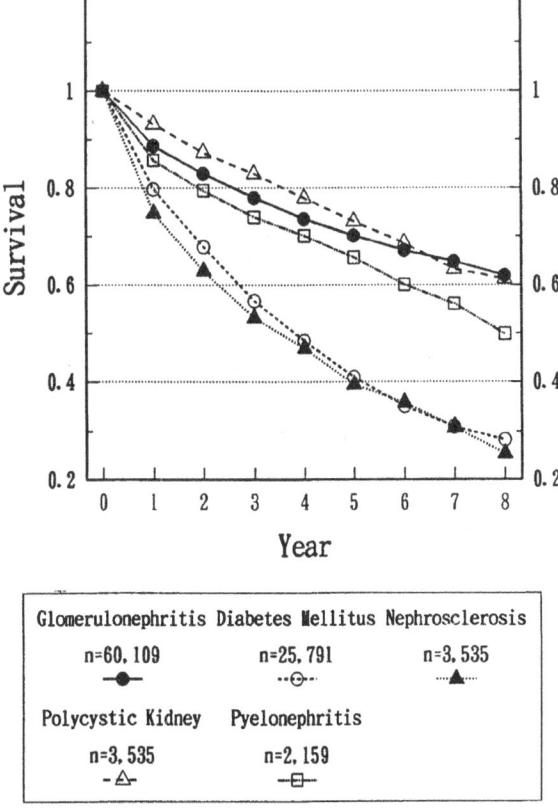

Fig. 5. Cumulative survival by original diseases in Japan in 131,585 ESRD patients who started dialysis after 1983.

Mortality

Per cent gross mortality in 1991 calculated by the consensus and the number of deaths was 8.85% and not different from those in recent eight years. Cumulative survival of 123,668 ESRD patients who started dialysis after 1983 was 0.833 at one year, 0.698 at three years, 0.648 at five years, and 0.523 at eight years.

Cumulative survivals analyzed by original diseases apparently showed a poor prognosis for DM and nephrosclerosis (Fig. 6).

The age, gender, serum creatinine concentrations, periods of start of dialysis (1983–1986 and 1987–1989), and original diseases were analyzed as prognostic markers by Cox's proportional hazard model. Table 1 shows significantly high hazard ratios for myeloma kidney, hereditary metabolic diseases, malignancy in the urinary tract, amyloid kidney, SLE, rapidly progressive glomerulonephritis, DM nephropathy, malignant hypertension, and nephrosclerosis.

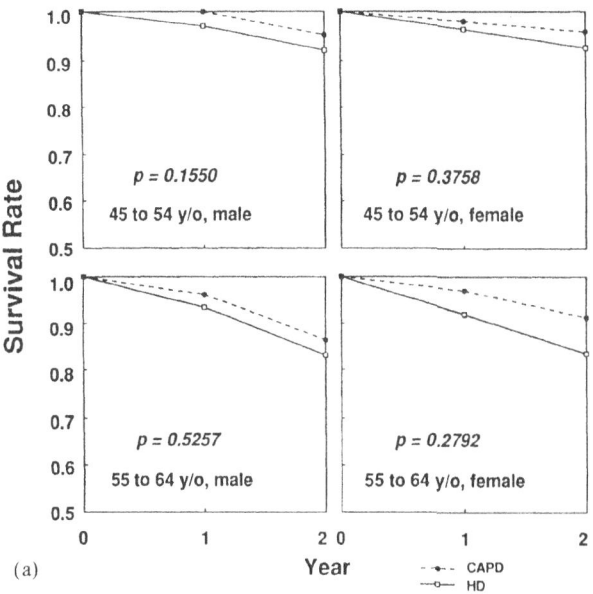

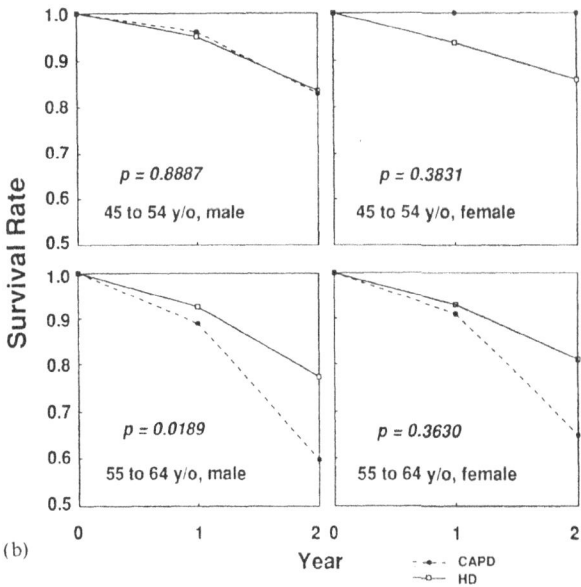

Fig. 6. Two-year survival of hemodialysis and CAPD patients by gender, age and original diseases. (a) Survival rates of dialysis patients without diabetes mellitus by modality ($n \times 5$, 081). (b) Survival rates of dialysis patients with diabetes mellitus by mortality ($n \times 1$, 906).

Table 1. Hazard ratios of mortality by original deceases in dialysis patients in Japan

Original disease	Hazard ratio 95%	Confidence range	P value
Chronic glomerulonephritis	1		
Chronic pyelonephritis	1.13	1.04–1.23	0.0025
Progressive glomerulonephritis	2.53	2.30–2.78	<0.0001
Toxemia	0.74	0.60–0.93	0.0092
Glomerulonephritis, unclassified	1.99	1.81–2.18	<0.0001
Polycystic kidney disease	0.84	0.78–0.90	<0.0001
Nephrosclerosis	1.38	1.31–1.44	<0.0001
Malignant hypertension	1.45	1.32–1.59	<0.0001
Diabetes mellitus	1.80	1.76–1.85	<0.0001
Systemic lupus erythematosus	2.79	2.53–3.08	<0.0001
Amyloid kidney	3.27	2.96–3.62	<0.0001
Hereditary metabolic diseases	3.50	3.21–3.82	<0.0001
Urinary tract tuberculosis	0.88	0.75–1.04	n.s.
Urolithiasis	0.95	0.79–1.14	n.s.
Malignancy in urinary tract	3.48	3.17–3.81	<0.0001
Obstructive uropathy	1.95	1.75–2.17	<0.0001
Myeloma kidney	4.47	3.97–4.81	<0.0001
Aplasia of kidneys	1.34	0.93–1.93	n.s.
Unknown origins	1.82	1.74–1.91	<0.0001

Each hazard ratio was calculated as the ratio to that of chronic glomerulonephritis with standardization by gender, age and period of start of dialysis therapy.

Patients were divided into three groups by serum creatinine concentrations of less than 5 mg/dl, less than 10 mg/dl and more than 10 mg/dl at the first dialysis therapy. Hazard ratios of groups with creatinine concentrations of less than 5 mg/dl and less than 10 mg/dl, compared with groups with creatinine concentrations of more than 10 mg/dl, were 2.35 (95% confidence range of 2.14–2.58, $p \times 0.0001$) and 1.54 (1.46–1.62, $p \times 0.0001$), respectively.

For international comparisons, survival rates at one year and two years are given in Fig. 6, arranged according to ages 45–54 and 55–65 years, gender, with/without diabetes, and treatment modalities.

Discussion

We described and analyzed our longitudinal survey data of dialysis therapy in Japan. Our longitudinal data clearly indicated that the mortality of dialysis patients in Japan depends on original diseases, creatinine concentration and age at the start of dialysis therapy. As noticed in world-wide surveys, DM and nephrosclerosis gave a poor prognosis for both hemodialysis and CAPD in Japan. The differences of survival were noted in two year survival curves of hemodialysis and CAPD patients in males and age group of 55–64 years old. The selection criteria of CAPD patients were not controlled because of a lack of this information. Difficulties in blood pressure control and constructing blood access might be the reasons of modality selection for CAPD. Those complications might accompany severe cardiac and vascular lesions, resulting in poor prognosis for CAPD patients.

The entry criteria to our survey were the start of dialysis therapy of ESRD patients, as in the EDTA and the Canadian survey; that was different from the criterion of the ninetieth day after the start of chronic dialysis used in the USRDS. The source of data was a questionnaire gathered by the JSDT Survey Committee with 95%–98% recovery. Confidence of the data depended on the personal reliability of those who filled out the questionnaire. In contrast, USRDS survey came from reliable financial records from dialysis facilities of Medicare-eligible patients in the Health Care Financial Administration, that covered 90% of ESRD patients.

Other than these differences in survey methods, there were many influencing factors, like age distribution of the population, differing races of patients, access to life-saving therapy, availability of hospitalization, or financial support for non-dialysis medical costs. These differences might make it difficult or meaningless to analyze international data to confirm medical determinants on mortality. The factors that were shown to be determinant candidates for dialysis mortality must be confirmed by well-controlled prospective study.

We will get more precise data about the survival and morbidity in the near future by longitudinal observations of those Japanese patients whose modalities and doses of dialysis therapy were determined in 1991. International comparisons with those Japanese data and those of other countries might give us valuable information concerning dialyzer-reuse, short-time dialysis, or effects of races on mortality, which might change the selection criteria for modality choices and prescription of ESRD therapy.

References

1. Alan R, Parker T. Proceedings from the mortality, morbidity and prescription of dialysis symposium, Dallas, Tx, September 15 to 17, 1989. Am J kidney disease 1990; 15: 75–383.
2. Alter M, Favero MS, Moyer LA, Bland LA. National surveillance of dialysis-associated diseases in the United States, 1989. Trans Am Soc Artif Intern Organs 1991; 37: 97–109.
3. Tufveson G, Geeling W, Broyer M, et al. EDTA registry center survey. Nephrol Dial Transplant 1989; 4: 161–171.
4. Held P, Levin NW, Bovbjerg RR, et al. Mortality and duration of hemodialysis treatment. JAMA 1991; 265: 871–875.
5. Levinsky NG, and Rettig RA. The Medicare end-stage renal disease program. A report from the Institute of Medicine. New Eng J Med 1991; 324(16): 1143–1148.
6. Rettig RA. Kidney failure and the federal government. The institute of medicine report on the Medicare End-Stage Renal Disease Program. AKF Nephrology Letters 1991; 3(3): 21–28.
7. Held P, Levin NW, Bovbjerg RR. Mortality and duration of hemodialysis treatment. JAMA 1991; 265: 871–875.
8. Joint Working Party on Diabetic Renal Failure of the British Diabetic Association. Treatment and mortality from diabetic renal failure in patients identified in the 1985 United Kingdom survey. Brit Med J 1989; 299: 1135–1136.
9. End-stage Renal Disease in New York State. Monograph series Number 1, School of Public Health University at Albany, State University of New York, New York State Department of Health, New York State, New York, 1991.

10. Odaka M. Annual Reports of the National Survey of Dialysis Therapy in Japan. The Survey Committee of Japanese Society for Dialysis Therapy, Chiba, Japan (in Japanese), 1983–1988.
11. Sawanishi K. Annual Report of the National Survey of Dialysis Therapy in Japan. The Survey Committee of Japanese Society for Dialysis Therapy, Nagoya, Japan (in Japanese), 1989
12. Maeda K. Annual Reports of the National Survey of Dialysis Therapy in Japan. The Survey Committee of Japanese Society for Dialysis Therapy, Nagoya, Japan (in Japanese) 1990–1991.
13. Akiba T, Kitaoka T, Kubo K, et al. Changes in the age distribution of chronic dialysis patients in Japan. J Jap Soc Dial Ther 1992; 25: 445–450 (in Japanese).
14. The Survey Committee of Japanese Society for Dialysis Therapy. The chronic dialysis patients registry in Japan–1991. Jap Soc Dial Ther 1991; 26: 17–30, 1993.
15. Gotch FA, Sargent JA A mechanistic analysis of the National Corporative Dialysis Study (NCDS). Kidney Int 1985; 28: 526–534.
16. Lowrie EG, Teehan BP Principles of prescribing dialysis therapy: Implementing recommendation from the National Cooperative dialysis Study. Kidney Int 1983; 23 (Suppl 13): S113–S122.

CHAPTER 6

International comparisons of dialysis survival are meaningless to evaluate differences in dialysis procedures

CARL M. KJELLSTRAND

Introduction

International comparisons of survival of dialysis patients have become popular [1–4]. Such comparisons have been used to evaluate differences in the procedure of hemodialysis. In general, the conclusions have been that short dialysis (independent of Kt/V values), low Kt/V values, the procedure of re-use of dialyzers, or non-compliance by patients, are responsible for the fact that survival is best in Japan, second-best in Europe, and lowest in the US [1–4]. There are many factors that influence mortality of dialysis patients (Table 1). Many are subjects of controversy even in single factor analyses. The interaction of many such factors is virtually unknown.

In this chapter I will argue that such international comparisons about the influence of dialysis technology on mortality are meaningless and that most of the differences can be explained by different patient populations and transplant rates. In the US, patients on dialysis are much older and have many and more severe co-morbid conditions and thus, naturally will have shorter survival than patients in Europe. The transplant rate in the US is very high, removing those who would have survived a long time on dialysis to transplantation. The transplant rate in Japan is only one-tenth of that in the US, and explains much of the very good survival rate of dialysis patients there [1–9]. To caricaturize this, a hardhearted nephrologist who excludes the sick and old from dialysis and then does not transplant the young and healthy always shows better survival rates than one who generously accepts old and sick patients and transplants many patients, independent of the dialysis technology used.

Secondly, to bolster my argument I will point out that Europe is not a country but a continent, and that the mortality rate on dialysis shows a great variation, being highest in the Scandinavian countries and lowest in Latin Europe (Italy, Spain and France), not because dialysis is better in Latin Europe than in Scandinavia, but because of differences in selection and trans-

55

E. A. Friedman (ed.), Death on Hemodialysis, 55–68.
© 1994 *Kluwer Academic Publishers.*

Table 1. Risk factors for death in dialysis patients

	I. PRE-EXISTING	
1.	*Demographic*	
	Age	XXX
	Sex	O
	Race	XX
2.	*Social*	
	Married	?
	Family support	?
	Area	?
	Smoking	?
	Alcohol	?
	Income	?
3.	*Diagnosis*	
	Diabetes	XXX
	Hypertensive nephrosclerosis	XX
	Systemic disease	XX
	Polycystic kidney disease	++
4.	*Type and duration of renal failure*	
	Acute	?
	Intermediate	?
	Chronic	?
	Late start	XX
5.	*Comorbid conditions*	
	Chronic heart failure	XXX
	Arteriosclerotic heart disease	XXX
	Stroke	XXX
	Peripheral vascular disease	?
	Pulmonary	XXX
	Malignancy	XXX
	Gastro-intestinal	?
	Hepatic	?
	Hypertension	XX
	II. SELECTION	
6.	Generous acceptance	XXX
	High transplant rate	XXX

plantation practice: the Scandinavians accept more patients and have a very high transplant rate, and have the worst dialysis patient survival in Europe [9–10]. Thirdly, the presently used proportional hazards analysis statistics are not adequate when comparing patient populations with wide discrepancies in age.

My final argument will be that unless there are more than trivial differences in survival between short and long dialysis and between re-use and non re-use, short dialysis with reuse by making dialysis cheaper and more effective makes it available to many more patients. Clearly, the US has 'won' the race for dialysis. In 1990 215 patients per million population (pmp) began dialysis

Table 1. (continued)

	III. TREATMENT RELATED	
7.	Late start	XX
	Insufficient (Kt/V <0.90?)	XXX
	IPD	XXX
	CAPD	?
	Fast dialysis	?
	Blood pressure control	XXX
	Biocompatibility	?
	Water quality	?
	Membrane type (open vs close)	?
	Reuse	?X
8.	*Patient*	
	Malnutrition (low BUN/CR-ratio low BUN, low cholesterol low ALB, low BMI, low transferrin)	XXX
	High CA × PO$_4$ product	XXX
	High interdialytic weight gain	XXX
	Inactivity	XXX
	Blood pressure control	XXX
	High creatinine	++

XXX Leads to higher mortality
O   Of no influence on mortality
++   Leads to lower mortality
?   Influence unknown

there, while the mean acceptance rate for Europe was only 48 pmp, less than a quarter of that in US, and only one European country, Austria, at that time had even broken through the 100/million population/year range. It is better to save 215 patients for 5 years (1075 patient years) than 48 patients for 10 years (480 patient years). For 1990 three times as many transplants (approximately 40 pmp) were done in US as in Europe (17 pmp) [5, 9].

Selection sets the stage for mortality

The selection of patients is important in determining what mortality rates one experiences. Figure 1 outlines the acceptance rates per year per million over the last 20 years in several countries in Europe, Japan and North America. In the US, more than twice as many patients are accepted as in the most generous countries in Europe, and 50% more patients than in Japan. Within Europe there are large variations in acceptance rates between 40 per million population in the UK, to Austria at 105 per million population per year, the most generous country in Europe for accepting patients. The mean age of acceptance is also much higher in the US, 64 years of age compared to less than 60 years of age in any European country [1–10]. It can be thought that these age differences are trivial but they are not. This is for two reasons, one dealing with the co-morbidity, the other one with the biological fact of death curves.

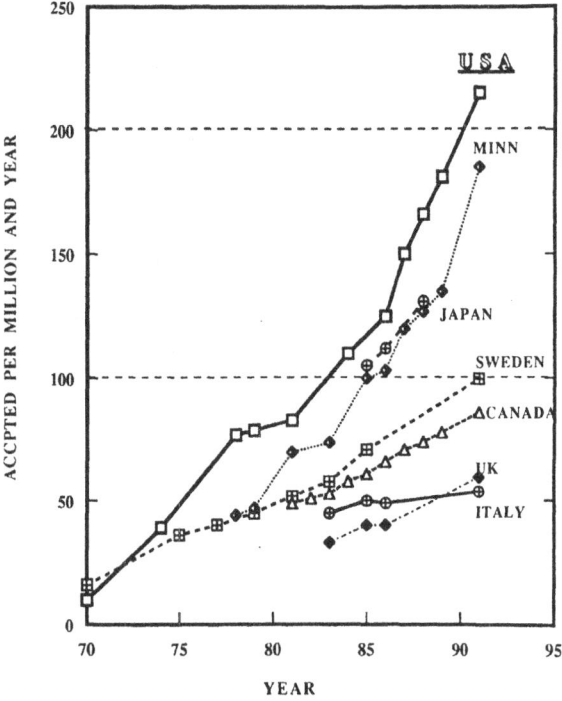

Fig. 1.   Acceptance rate per million population/year in US, Japan and several European countries. US is taking more than twice as many patients as any European country and 50% more patients than in Japan.

Acceptance and co-morbidity

Figure 2 illustrates how the patient population has changed at a large US centre over 20 years of dialysis. Already in the mid and late 60s all patients below age 50 without co-morbidity were accepted and this patient group has not increased since. In the mid 70's there was a large increase in the young patients with complications, basically because dialysis was started on diabetic patients at that time. At approximately the same time older patients without any co-morbidity were accepted. Since 1976 the only group that has shown an increase are the old patients with considerable co-morbidity [11]. Clearly, co-morbidity and disease increase stepwise and are not proportional to acceptance rates. These old patients are the ones still left untreated in Europe; comparison of acceptance patterns of patients to dialysis in Stockholm and Minneapolis shows that clearly [11–13].

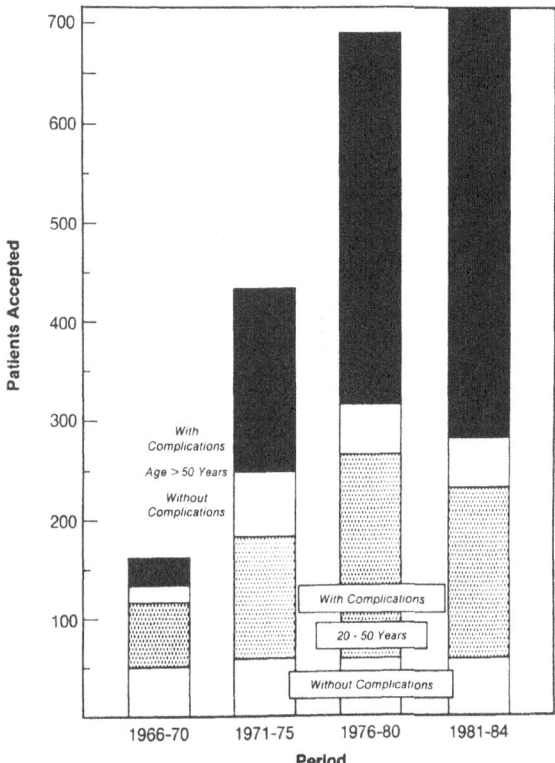

Fig. 2. Characteristics of changes in the patient population over 20 years in a large US dialysis centre. Already in the late 60s, all young patients without co-morbid conditions and complications were accepted and that patient group has not increased since. In the early 70s young patients with complications, mainly consisting of diabetic patients, and patients above age 50 without complications were accepted and since then there has been virtually no increase in these patient groups. The only patient group that has increased and that remains to be treated are in the old patients with many other diseases. This characteristic of changes in patient populations over time makes hazards non-proportional even when correcting for age. (Figure from [11]. Reprinted with permission of Springer-Verlag.)

Transplantation and co-morbidity

Organs for transplantation are a scarce commodity and even in countries that recruit the most donors, transplantation is the exception. Most patients who start dialysis will remain on it till their deaths. Naturally, the transplant surgeons select the patients with the longest survival probability, i.e. the young and those without co-morbid conditions. In one study, dialysis patients who went on to transplantation had less than half the number of comorbid conditions when compared to those who remained on dialysis [14, 15]. Thus, generous transplant rates adversely affect the survival curves on dialysis.

Patients with long survival potential are chosen for transplantation, leaving those with only short survival prognosis on dialysis. This explains much of the superior survival of dialysis patients in Japan which has a transplant rate only one-tenth of that in the US [5, 8]. Similarly, the transplant rate in the US is three times that in Europe as a conglomerate, 40 vs 17 pmp per year. Only five countries could match the US, and two of these were in Scandinavia (Norway and Sweden).

Analysis of the effect of acceptance and transplant rates on dialysis survival

An analysis of differences in mortality between 5 European regions and the US as dependent on acceptance rates and transplant rates is shown in Fig. 3 [9–13]. It is clear that the R values are high. When the data were subjected to stepwise and multiple regression analysis:

4 year cumulative dialysis survival =

$100 - 0.17 \times$ acceptance rate of patients per million population $- 0.4 \times$ percent transplanted at 4 years $+ 7$

$R = 0.96, P = 0.02$

Thus, in this particular analysis, over 90% of the differences in cumulative survival between five European regions and the US were explained by different acceptance and transplant rates even in age matched patients. We are presently analyzing this separately for older patients and also in patients with diabetes. Thus, not more than 10% of differences in mortality rates between different regions of Europe and the US can be due to factors other than selection or transplantation. The lesson is clear, the hardhearted nephrologist who does not accept the old and the sick and then in addition does not transplant, is going to show good survival rates. Undoubtedly, many of the supreme survival results of dialysis in Japan are simply due to the fact that the young and the healthy do not undergo transplantation there, as in other parts of the world, but remain for decades of dialysis.

Errors in analysis of mortality

Dialysis mortality is presently analyzed using conventional and correct cumulative survival. This is further analyzed by the Proportional Hazards model described by Cox [16].

These models assume some form of similarity between the shapes of the cumulative survival curves and thus some proportionality that remains constant when correcting for different risk factors. These assumptions are incorrect. Figure 4 illustrates the general 'ideal' death curve. Many countries have now come very close to having this shape. However, the exact location of the curve varies considerably. For example, the mean life expectancy at birth is now the longest in Japan, being 79 years for a man, 4 years more than

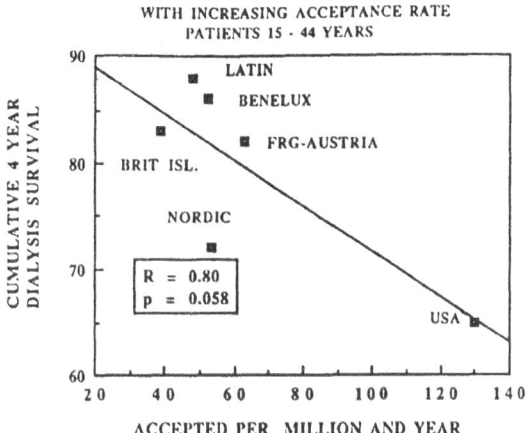

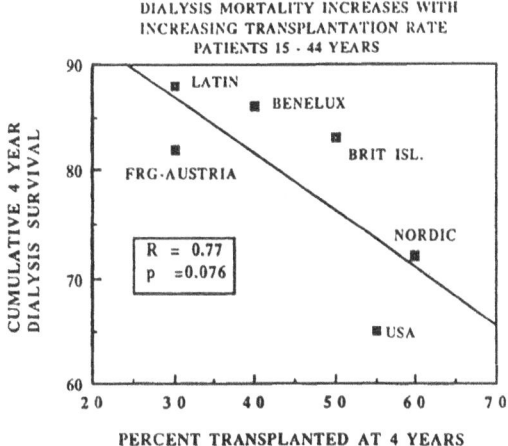

Fig. 3.   Simple linear regression analysis relating dialysis mortality to patients accepted per million/year in 5 different European regions and the US and setting dialysis mortality in relation to transplant rates in the same geographical areas. There are quite high R values suggesting that both acceptance rates and transplant rates are responsible for much of the differences in mortality between different areas. Latin Europe (France, Italy and Spain) have the best survival rates but also accept the fewest patients and have done very few transplants. On the contrary the worst survival is found in the Nordic countries (Denmark, Norway, Sweden and Finland) and the US. But these regions also accept many more patients and transplant at a much higher rate than the other areas. If one does a multiple regression analysis, the R = 0.96 and the P = <0.02, taking into consideration both acceptance and transplant rates, suggesting that over 90% of the difference in mortalities can be explained by these factors alone. Clearly, acceptance and transplant rates dwarf other factors influencing differences in mortality studies such as re-use and short dialysis. (Figure reprinted from [12] with permission of W. B. Saunders Co.)

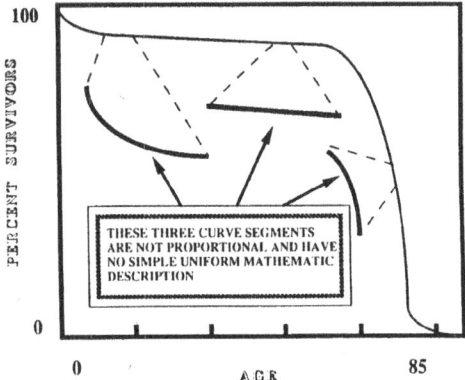

Fig. 4. The general and ideal mortality curve. There is some mortality in the newborns but from then on very low mortality rates are encountered until approximately age 70 where the survival falls off steeply. Clearly, the shape of the curve is different depending on age, and as a patient group ages the mortality curve is undergoing a complicated change that cannot be easily described mathematically.

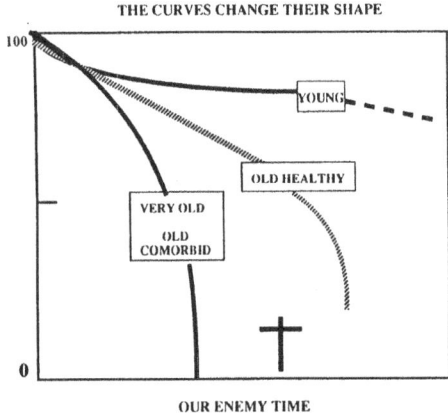

Fig. 5. Mortality curves for different patient groups on dialysis. These curves are not parallel and within each group change with time.

in the US, life expectancy there being 75 years of age. One can thus assume that in particular, older dialysis patients of the same age would show a better survival in Japan than in the US.

The second observation is that the curve changes shape. It is concave for the newborn and the young, approximately straight for the young to middle-aged, then becomes steeply convex for the old, ultimately having a slight concavity for the extreme ages (Fig. 4). If one looks at ideal survival curves of patients on dialysis on Fig. 5 it is clear that first the curves have a different

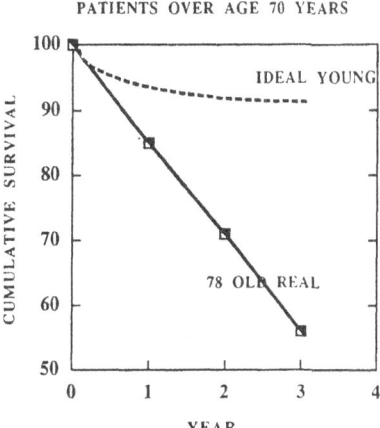

Fig. 6.   The actual mortality curve for 78 very old dialysis patients. These patients were all above age 70 years, the mean age was 75 years. These patients were prospectively analyzed and followed for three years. No-one was withdrawn to transplantation or lost to follow up. Unlike the exponential curves, usually found for other patient populations, the survival curve falls in a straight line, bolstering the argument made in the legend to Fig. 5. The shape of the mortality curve is different in different age groups and constantly changes for a given group of patients.

shape, the young concave curve is ultimately becoming straight, the straight curve for the old and healthy will become concave and it will be steeply concave for the very old and the old who have a co-morbid condition. There is no proportionality and there is no easy mathematical solution to describe these curves, nor are they proportional. That this is in fact true is illustrated in Fig. 6 in which survival of young patients is compared to that actually found in patients over the age of 70 years [17]. None of the old patients were 'censored', all were followed till death or endpoint. Obviously the older patient has a straight mortality curve, something that common sense would have dictated as opposed to the presently used logarithmic appearance of survival curves found in younger dialysis patients. The latter assumes that some dialysis patient will be immortal, which is highly unlikely.

Figure 7 illustrates the percentage of dialysis patients who are between age 65 and 74 years and 75<plus> years in Europe, erroneously regarded as a conglomerate and the US. Obviously the patients on dialysis in the US are much older than those who receive treatment in Europe. This will increase the mortality risk of US patients in a non-proportional way. First of all the shape of the curves will change, secondly there will be many more co-morbid conditions in US patients. These factors are synergistic in increasing mortality in an unknown way [18].

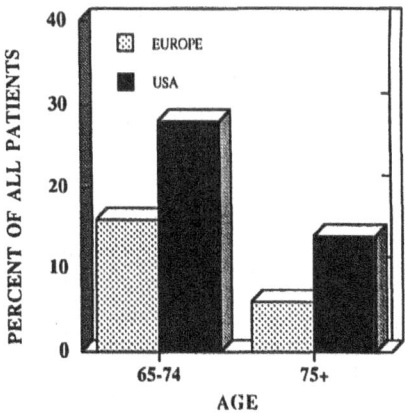

Fig. 7. Percent of patients in the US and Europe that were between 64 years of age or above 75 years of age in Europe and the US. Twice as many patients in the US between 65 and 74 years are started on dialysis pmp per year as in Europe and there are three times as many patients started on dialysis above 75 years in the US when compared to Europe.

Other investigators have also come to the conclusion that proportional hazards analysis is not adequate when describing those who are very old or very sick [19, 20].

Analysis of the influence of adequacy, speed and reuse on dialysis mortality

There are many problems in these analyses. Each of them is obviously worthy of evaluation, however many of these factors, and reuse in particular, will probably have, if any, only a small influence on mortality, and it certainly will be dwarfed by geographical differences in patient selection and other treatment factors as outlined in Table 1. The only way to analyze such a small influence is by prospective randomized studies.

Adequacy

The only thorough analysis of adequacy is that of the National Cooperative Dialysis Study by Gotch [21, 22]. Gotch's original conclusion was that there was a stepwise increment in morbidity and mortality once adequacy, defined as Kt/V in three times a week dialysis, fell below 1. This assumption has since been challenged and Charra in particular believes the value should be much higher, probably even above 1.6 [3]. There are many problems with Charra's approach in that Charra analyzed young, non-diabetic patients who then did not receive a transplant. The relative mortality rate in patients treated by Charra and those in the US is illustrated in Fig. 8 [3, 5]. Clearly the survival of Charra's patients is spectacular when compared to that in the US. The selection

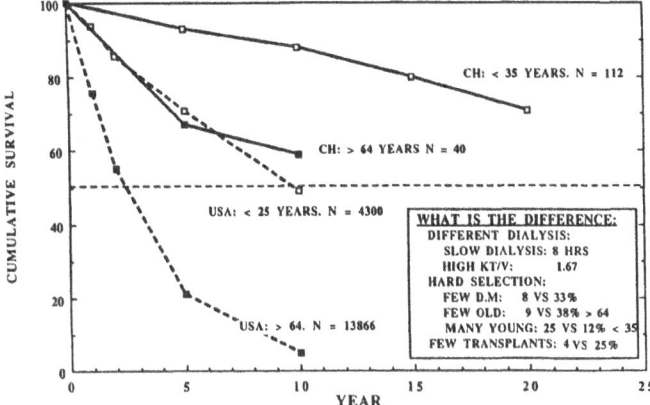

Fig. 8. Survival curves from the US RDS book and Charra's Kidney International article [3, 5]. The survival is spectacular in Charra's patients and much better than that experienced in the US even when patients are approximately of similar age. However, it is clear that Charra's patients were much more selected than in the US. In the US there are three times as many patients above age 64 as below age 25, there is only one-third as many patients over age 64 or below even 35 in Charra's series. There are four times more patients with diabetes mellitus in the US than in Charra's series and the transplant rate in the US is 6 times that of Charra's patients. This hard selection and absence of transplantation certainly explains much of the very fine survival seen by Charra and his group, and to assign the superior survival to slow dialysis and high Kt/V is impossible.

used is also listed in Fig. 8. Clearly, Charra's patients are younger, have less diabetes and a very small chance of undergoing transplantation. These selection factors probably contribute much more to the improved survival rates than the fact that dialysis by Charra was longer, slower and with a much higher Kt/V than in the US.

The same critique applies to his own data that show that patients dialysed with a Kt/V more than 1.6 (the mean of the group) survived better than those who were dialyzed with a Kt/V of < 1.6. The group with a higher Kt/V were more often women, were younger and had better blood pressure control. It is thus impossible to sort out exactly which of these factors was responsible for the better survival as no multifactorial analysis, with all its uncertainties, was even attempted [3].

Open membranes

A recent study found that a group of patients treated with high flux dialysis had better survival than those treated with conventional dialysis [23]. However, the same critique discussed above applies to this study in that patients on conventional dialysis were 4 years older, were more often male and white, and more often had diabetes, hypertension, cardiovascular disease, peptic ulcer disease and malignancy, as well as a considerably lower admission albumen.

Although a multi-factorial proportional hazards analysis was applied and indicated that open membrane carried a superior survival, the problem is that proportional hazards were probably not proportional as discussed above.

Reuse of dialyzers

Reuse of dialyzers is often practised in the US, less often in Europe, and almost not at all in Japan [1, 2, 4–10]. Thus, the practice of reuse and mortality are in parallel and it has been argued that reuse is one factor responsible for the high mortality in US. There are many errors in the reasoning, and Levin has recently raised some of those counter-arguments [24]. The question of the effects of reuse on mortality simply cannot be answered by comparing survival rates, even in age matched patients from different countries. If reuse has an influence, it is probably trivial and has to be analyzed within an institution and in a prospective randomized study, not by comparing survival in one country to other with other factors which almost certainly dwarf any of the possible advantage of non-reuse.

A utilitarian consideration

What if reuse and fast dialysis lead to slightly worse survival? Obviously it has by no means been proven that either reuse or fast dialysis are particularly dangerous but it is not unreasonable to speculate that they are. One thing is certain and that is if fast dialysis is used and if reuse is applied on a sound financial basis, with the same amount of money, personnel and time, one can treat many more patients than if one does not reuse, or if one uses very long and slow dialyses or expensive equipment.

In the US more than twice as many patients are put on dialysis as any country in Europe and in most instances four times as many patients are being started yearly per million population. The acceptance rate to dialysis in the US is 50% is higher than in Japan.

From pure utilitarian reasoning it appears better to save 215 patients for 5 years than 48 patients for 10 years. With that reasoning, in the US 1075 patient years would be gained versus only 480 in Europe. Clearly, such economic and organizational factors must be considered. It is also extremely unlikely that either re-use or fast dialysis would double mortality, as used in this example. It is simply used to bring some form of common sense utilitarianism into the debate. Rather than bragging of a year or two longer survival it appears that Europeans would do well to consider taking care of more old patients than they presently do rather than letting them die from uremia. In the overall affairs of a uremic population, it is clear that the US has offered dialysis treatment to more of those at risk than any country in the world [1–10, 25].

Summary

Niggardly selection and niggardly transplant rates are the factors that make dialysis survival appear good on paper, more so than the contribution of either reuse or fast dialysis to decreased survival rates. International comparisons ignoring these selection factors and attributing difference in survival to technique, are meaningless. Pure utilitarian reasoning suggests that fast dialysis and reuse are important determinants in how many patients can be treated in a country with a given budget. With the present economic circumstances being harsh even in the most rich countries, it would be foolish to ignore such factors particularly when based on international survival comparison. The presently used mortality statistics are also flawed when used for proportional hazards analysis.

References

1. Held PJ, Blagg CR, Liska DW, Port FK, Hakim R, Levin N. The dose of hemodialysis according to dialysis prescription in Europe and the United States. Kid Int 1992; 42 (Suppl 38): S16–S21.
2. Brunner, FP, Selwood NH. Profile of patients on RRT in Europe and death rates due to major causes of death groups. Kid Int 1992; 42 (Suppl 38): S14–S15.
3. Charra, B, Calemard E, Ruffet M, Chazot C, Terrat JC, Vanel T, Laurent G. Survival as in index of adequacy of dialysis. Kid Int 1992; 41: 1286–1291.
4. Shaldon S. Adequacy of long-term hemodialysis. Current Opinion in Nephrology and Hypertension 1992; 1: 197–202.
5. US Renal Data System, USRDS 1991 Annual Data Report, The National Institutes of Health, National Institute of Diabetes and Digestive and Kidney Diseases, Bethesda, MD August 1990.
6. Canadian Organ Replacement Register 1990 Annual Report, Hospital Medical Records Institute, Don Mills, Ontario, March 1992.
7. Combined report on regular dialysis and transplantation in Europe, IX, 1978. Proceedings of the European Dialysis and Transplant Association 1979; The Netherlands: London: Pitman Medical, 1979.
8. Japanese Dialysis Registry 1985, 1986, 1988. Tokyo, Japan.
9. Report on management of renal failure in Europe, XXII, 1991. Nephrol Dial Transplant 1992; 7 (Suppl 2).
10. Report from the European Dialysis and Transplant Association Registry: Demography of dialysis and transplantation in Europe in 1985 and 1986: Trends over the previous decade. Nephrol Dial Transplant 1988; 3: 714–727.
11. Kjellstrand CM, Matson M. Demand for and changing patient population, mortality, and death patterns in chronic dialysis. In: HJ Gurland, editor. Uremia Therapy. Berlin Heidelberg: Springer-Verlag, 1987: 218–243.
12. Kjellstrand CM, Hylander B, Collins AC. Mortality on dialysis – on the influence of early start, patient characteristics, and transplantation and acceptance rates. Am J Kid Dis 1990; 5: 483–490.
13. Hylander, B, Lunblad H, Kjellstrand CM. Changing patient characteristics in chronic hemodialysis. Scand J Urol Nephrol 1991; 25: 59–63.
14. Jacobson SH, Fryd D, Sutherland DER, Kjellstrand CM. Treatment of the diabetic patient with end-stage renal failure. Diabetes/Metabolism/Reviews 1988; 4: no. 3: 191–200.
15. Matson M, Kjellstrand CM. Long-term follow up of 369 diabetic patients undergoing dialysis. Arch Intern Med 1988; 148: 600–604.

16. Cox DR. Regression models and lifte tables. Journal of the Royal Statistical Society Series B, 34, 187–220, 1972.
17. Husebye DG, Westlie L, Styrvoky TJ, Kjellstrand CM. Psychological, social, and somatic prognostic indicators in old patients undergoing long-term dialysis. Arch Intern Med 1987; 147: 1921–1924.
18. Shapiro F, Umen A. Risk factors in hemodialysis patient survival. ASAIO J 1982; 6: 176–184.
19. Deeg DJH, Van Oortmarssen GJ, Habbema JDF, Van Der Maas PJ. A measure of survival time for long-term follow-up studies of the elderly. J Clin Epidemol 1989; 42: 541–549.
20. Wickramaratne PJ, Prusoff BA, Merikangas KR, Weissman MM. The use of survival time models with nonproportional hazard functions to investigate age of onset in family studies. J Chron Dis 1986; 39: 389–397.
21. Lowrie EG, Laird NM, Parker TF, Sargent JA. Effect of the hemodialysis prescription on patient morbidity. New Engl J Med 1981; 305: 1176–1181.
22. Gotch FA, Sargent JA. A mechanistic analysis of the National Cooperative Dialysis Study (NCDS). Kid Int 1985; 28: 526–534.
23. Hornberger JC, Chernew M, Petersen J, Garber AM. A multivariate analysis of mortality and hospital admissions with high-flux dialysis. J Am Soc Nephrol 1992; 3: 1227–1237.
24. Levin NW. Dialyzer Reuse: a currently acceptable practice. Seminars in Dialysis 1993; 6: 89–90.
25. Kjellstrand CM, Hasinoff D. Exclusion of old dialysis patients in the USA, Canada and Sweden. In: Oreopoulos DG, Michelis MF, Herschorn, editors. Nephrology and Urology in the Aged. Kluwer Acad Publishers, Netherlands 1993, pp. 569–583.

CHAPTER 7

Peracetic acid reuse as a risk factor for hemodialysis patient survival

ALLAN J. COLLINS, JENNIE MA and ANDREW UMEN

Introduction

The practice of reuse of hemodialyzers within the United States has been increasing more rapidly since the introduction in 1982 of the composite rate for reimbursement for dialysis [1,2]. Concerns about the procedural aspects of reuse led to the development of recommended practices for reuse by the American Association for Medical Instrumentation (AAMI). These guidelines have been incorporated into federal regulations for dialysis providers [2,3]. During the same interval of time as reuse was increasing from 1982 to 1988, the one-, two-, and five-year survival data of US patients was not improving compared to the same interval for European patients [4,5,6,7,8,9,10,11]. The survival of European patients was considerably better by as much as 20% compared to the United States data. Many factors have been proposed as explanations for the difference in the survival which included case mix, co-morbidity, and more recently, dialysis treatment time, delivered dialysis, and reuse of dialyzers [12,13,14,15,16]. Several studies have shown that the case mix in Europe may be different than in the United States, since the incidence of new end-stage renal disease patients is 3 to 3.5 times higher in the United States. More recently, the United States Renal Data System (USRDS) case mix study showed lower prescribed therapy within the United States compared to Europe, providing more concrete data which has been shown to impact on survival [4].

The issues of comparing results from different registries is confounded by the complexities of case mix and therapy differences as well as the issue of reuse, such that these factors are not evaluatable within the registries. In October of 1992, an FDA alert was issued after a reuse study sponsored by the Health Care Finance Administration (HCFA) showed an increased relative risk of death associated with two germicides, glutaraldehyde and peracetic acid, compared to no reuse in freestanding dialysis units using low-flux dialyzers [17]. The studies demonstrated an association of increased

E. A. Friedman (ed.), Death on Hemodialysis, 69–81.
© 1994 *Kluwer Academic Publishers.*

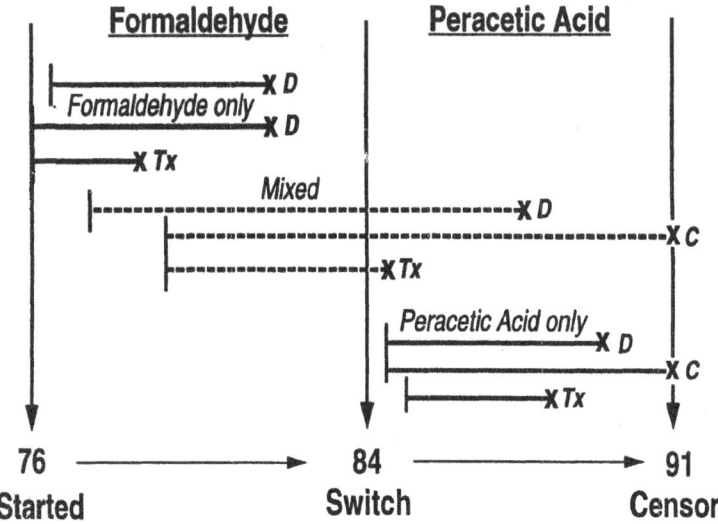

Fig. 1. Schematics of patient entry in the formaldehyde and peracetic acid time intervals. The time-dependent Cox regression analysis evaluates the survival time under each reuse agent. Key: D = death; Tx = transplant; C = censored.

mortality, but no hypothesis for the association was advanced, and no cause-specific death rates were affected which might provide a mechanism for the association. One of the major drawbacks of the HCFA study centered on the lack of detailed data on co-morbidity, dialysis therapy, and serum albumin levels, as well as the reuse procedures practiced throughout the United States. The reuse practices would include the type of reuse machines and concentrations of the germicides as well as compliance with AAMI reuse guidelines. To help evaluate these factors, the Regional Kidney Disease Program initiated a retrospective analysis of hemodialysis patient survival from 1976 to 1989, with follow-up through September 15, 1991. During this time interval, two forms of reuse were practiced: 2% to 4% formaldehyde from 1976 to 1983, and 3.5% peracetic acid from 1984 to the present [18]. We used a Cox time-dependent model to test whether survival of hemodialysis patients was affected by the change to peracetic acid reuse in 1984 after adjusting for primary renal diagnosis, diabetes, urea index (Kt/V), hypoalbuminemia, and clinical co-morbidity. This report summarizes the results of the analysis.

Methods

Patients entering hemodialysis from 1976 to 1989 with complete data sets on Kt/V and albumins were used for the analysis, which included 1,773 patients (1082 non-diabetics and 691 diabetics). Patients were classified by primary renal diagnosis, assessed for seven co-morbid conditions on entry to hemodialysis (atherosclerotic heart disease, congestive heart failure, other cardiac diseases, peripheral vascular disease, cancer, cerebrovascular accident, and chronic obstructive pulmonary disease) and defined as Type I or Type II diabetes based on ketosis-prone status. Dialysis therapy was quantitated by review of quarterly flow sheets for actual treatment time, blood flow rate, dialysate flow rate, dry weight, intradialytic weight loss, and patient height. Urea index was calculated from *in vitro* dialyzer clearances tested in our laboratory, the actual treatment time and blood flow rate from the dialysis flowsheet, and the volume of urea distribution by a sex/weight/height/age nomogram [19]. Each patient's quarterly Kt/V was averaged over the survival of the patient and used as a risk factor. Serum albumin on a quarterly basis was also averaged over the survival of the patient and used as a risk factor. Figure 1 shows the schematic of patient survival based on the year of entry and the 1984 switch year from formaldehyde to peracetic acid. Since the change to peracetic acid occurred during a time after the initiation of dialysis in many patients who survived to the switch year 1984, a time-dependent Cox regression analysis was used to evaluate not only the impact of the patient-specific risk factors but also the survival time on each reuse agent (formaldehyde and peracetic acid).

Patients were divided into diabetic and non-diabetic groups for analysis, since diabetic patients violate the proportionality assumptions of the Cox analysis [20]. The reference population for the non-diabetic patients was glomerulonephritis, non-hypertension, and non-paraprotein or renovascular renal disease. The reference population for diabetics was Type II diabetes. Both reference groups used patients aged 61 to 75 years, Kt/V $\pm$ 1.2 in non-diabetics, and $\pm$ 1.4 in diabetics, with an albumin $>$ 3.5 gm/dl. Statistical software used was BMDP 386 for the 486–50 mHz IBM computers and BMDP for the Vax 6000–610 Digital Equipment Corporation computer. An additional parameter included in the Cox analysis was the percentage of survival time on each reuse agent for the three patient types: formaldehyde only, mixed formaldehyde-peracetic acid, and peracetic acid only. Survival endpoints included death, censor for transplant, censor for change to another dialysis program, or censor at the follow-up date of September 15, 1991. Only first-time hemodialysis patients were used.

Reuse practices were evaluated by dialyzer testing under reuse with cuprophan dialyzers, which had been previously published for formaldehyde and peracetic acid reuse in the pre–1986 period [18]. In the high-efficiency era, CA 210 dialyzers (Baxter Healthcare Corporation, McGaw Park, Illinois) were evaluated at first and eighteenth reuse for urea and creatinine clearance under peracetic acid reuse in an *in vitro* system previously described. Clearances were performed at 400 ml/min blood flow rate and at 700 ml/min dialysate flow. Six dialyzers were tested in January of 1990 with random retesting during later periods showing the same results.

To determine if reuse practices for water were within the AAMI-recommended guidelines, the water treatment system basic design was outlined, and water

Table 1. RKDP reuse program

Dialyzer		Sterilant	No. reuse
66–74	Kills	Formaldehyde	–
75–83	Hollow fibers (cupraphan)	Formaldehyde	6–8
83–85	Hollow fibers (cupraphan)	Peracetic acid	6–8
86–92	Hollow fibers (cellulose acetate)	Peracetic acid	12–14

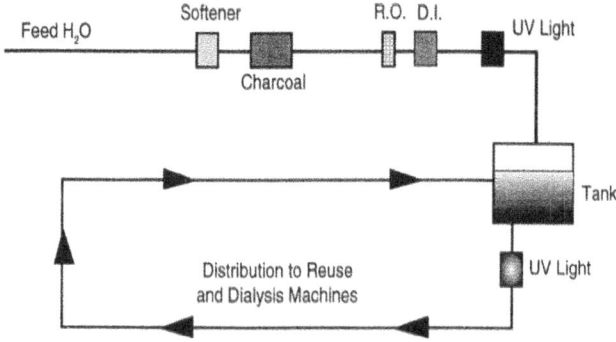

Fig. 2.   Schematic of the typical water treatment and distribution systems in the seven RKDP metropolitan dialysis units. Key: RO = Reverse osmosis; DI = deionization tanks; UV = ultraviolet lights.

cultures and endotoxin levels were retrospectively summarized. Unfortunately, only 6 months of data was on-line in the data base for review from October of 1992 to March of 1993. All water cultures were performed using a spread plate technique on standard methods media. Microbiologic evaluation under bicarbonate dialysate used tryptic soy agar. Endotoxin levels were measured by limulus amebocyte lysate testing using kits from Cape Cod Associates. Other clinical practices which were performed but not analyzed for this study included access recirculation and residual renal function studies every six months on all patients since 1986. The reuse procedures have been previously described up to 1984, with peracetic acid reuses performed with Renatron<reg> automated reprocessing equipment achieving a 3.25 % to 3.5 % concentration of peracetic acid in the dialyzer. All dialyzers were rinsed for 20 minutes with reverse osmosis water in the dialysate compartment in a reuse area since 1988 and primed with normal saline prior to patient use.

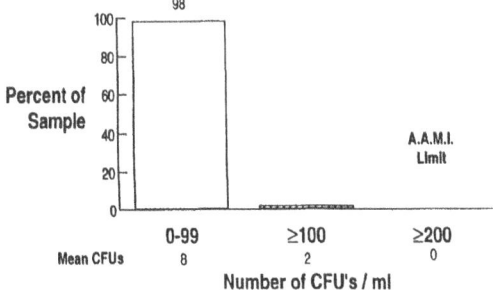

Fig. 3. Water system cultures on standard methods medium showing 98% of all cultures have a mean colony forming units per ml (CFUs) of 8 (N = 241).

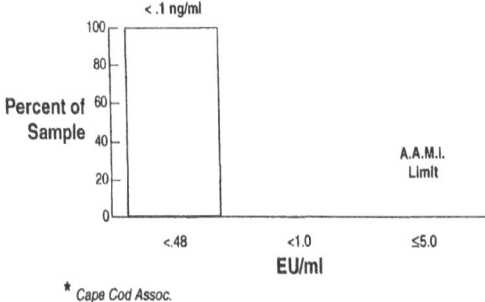

Fig. 4. Water system endotoxin levels as measured by a limulus amebocyte lysate test. The detection limits were 0.48 endotoxin units per ml. or less than 0.1 mg/ml. All tests were below the detector limits in water used for reuse and dialysate (N = 38).

Results

Table 1 shows the sequential history of the reuse program from formaldehyde to peracetic acid reuse in 1984. The mean number of reuses in the formaldehyde period was six to eight and was the same from 1984 to 1986, the pre-high-efficiency era [21,22,23,24]. High-efficiency CA 170 and CA 210 dialyzers (Baxter Healthcare Corporation, McGaw Park, Illinois) were used after 1986 with a mean of 12 to 14 reuses with peracetic acid. Figure 2 shows the basic water system design which supplies AAMI-quality water for dialysis and reuse. Note that each dialysis unit uses softeners to remove calcium and magnesium, charcoal to remove chlorine, chloramine, and nitrates, spiral-wound reverse osmosis units and followed by mixed-bed deionization tanks. Ultraviolet lights are used to control bacterial growth prior to the water entering a holding tank. The water is repressurized from the holding tank and distributed in a recirculating loop at five to seven gallons per minute with an additional ultraviolet light for bacterial control.

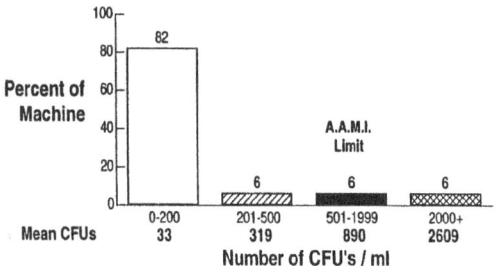

Fig. 5. Percent of dialysate machine cultures with the mean colony forming units per ml. Six percent of cultures exceeded the AAMI guidelines and required repeat bleach or peracetic acid sterilization (N = 700).

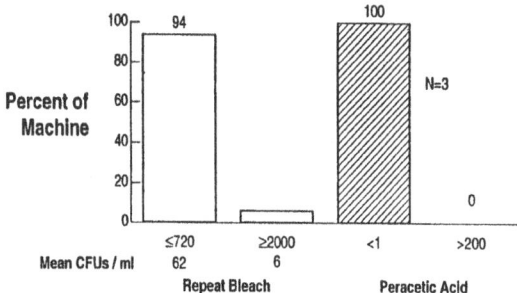

Fig. 6. The machines which initially exceeded the AAMI limits on repeat bleach sterilization. 94% of machines were within the culture limits. These machines required peracetic acid sterilization to finally reduce the CFUs and correct the contamination (N = 42).

Figures 3, 4, 5, and 6 show the results of cultures and endotoxin testing from the water systems for dialysis and reuse and the machine dialysate cultures. Ninety-eight percent of the 41 cultures had a mean colony count of 8 CFU per ml with 2 % of the cultures being between 100 CFU and less than 200 CFU per ml. No cultures were greater than 200 CFU per ml. Out of the 38 endotoxin samples tested in the seven dialysis units, all results were below the detection limits of less than 0.48 EU/ml, or < 0.1 ng/ml (AAMI recommended limits are ≤ 5.0 EU/ml). Dialysate cultures showed 82 % of machines had less than 200 CFU per ml (mean 33 CFU/ml). Six percent of machines had ± 2,000 colonies per ml which was resolved either by rebleaching the machines or with a singleperacetic acid sterilization as shown in Fig. 6.

In vitro testing of the CA 210 dialyzers is displayed in Fig. 7. Ninety-seven percent of urea and creatinine clearances were maintained after 18 peracetic acid reuses with no loss in the ultrafiltration coefficient (KUF).

Figure 8 shows the Cox regression analysis of the non-diabetic patients with no risks. The effect of age can be seen, although significance in this group was

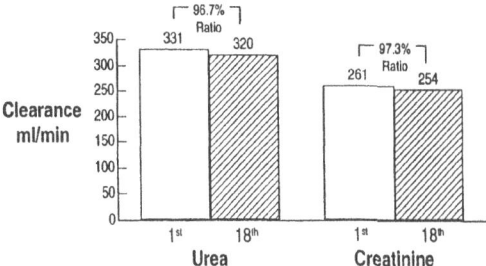

Fig. 7.   Comparison of the first and eighteenth reuse in initial clearances of urea and creatinine in CA 210 cellulose acetate dialyzers with 400 ml/min blood flow rates and 700 ml/min dialysate flow rates

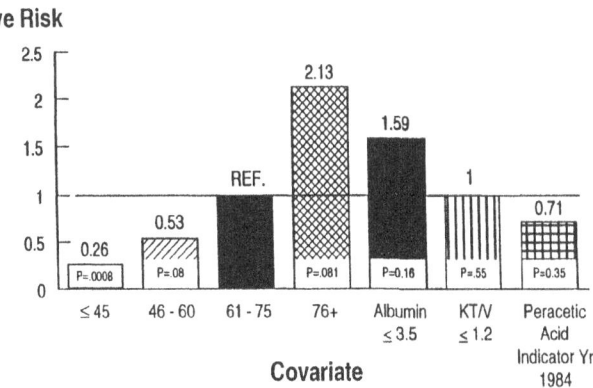

Fig. 8.   Cox regression analysis of 375 no-risk, non-diabetic patients. The baseline reference patients were non-diabetics with glomerulonephritis, a Kt/V ± 1.2, and an albumin > 3.5 gm/dl. (Formaldehyde reuse performed prior to 1984).

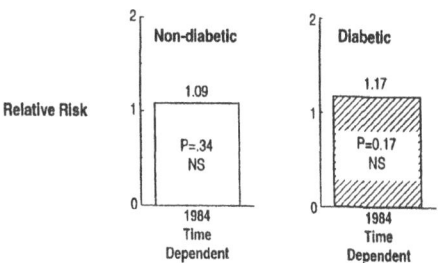

Fig. 9.   Cox time-dependent regression analysis of the relative risk of peracetic acid percent exposure compared to formaldehyde percent exposure with adjustments for age, renal diagnosis, diabetes Type I and Type II, and seven clinical co-morbid conditions only.

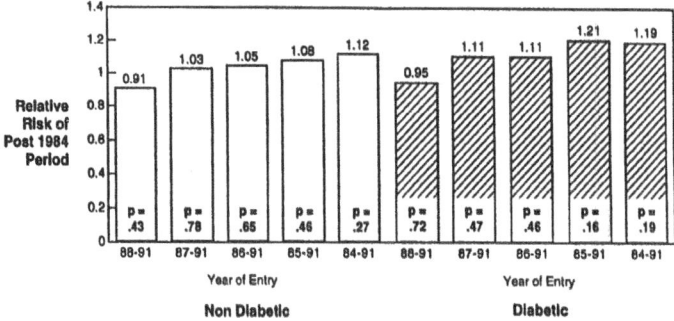

Fig. 10.   Cox regression analysis evaluating the year of entry of dialysis patients as a risk factor using 1984 as the indicator year, when peracetic acid reuse was introduced. As patients are added into the analysis from 1987 back to 1984, the direction of the relative risk changes, although significance was not achieved at a P-value of < 0.05.

not achieved secondary to the small sample size. The impact of a low albumin of ≤ 3.5 gm/dl is significant, but the effect of Kt/V ± 1.2 was not significant in this no-risk populations. Peracetic acid compared to formaldehyde was not a significant risk factor. Figure 9 shows the comparison of peracetic acid percent time exposure as a risk factor in all non-diabetic and diabetic patients. These results were adjusted for age, renal diagnosis, diabetes, and the seven co-morbid conditions. In both non-diabetic and diabetic patients, the time-dependent analysis shows the peracetic acid was not a significant risk factor, with P-values of 0.34 and 0.17, respectively.

Since the effect of the peracetic acid, although not significant, was in the direction of greater than 1.0 compared to formaldehyde, a further analysis was performed to determine if the year of entry impacted on the outcome of peracetic acid reuse since 1984. This was performed by comparing all formaldehyde patients from 1976 to 1983 with peracetic acid patients entering during the years 1988 to 1991, 1987 to 1991, 1986 to 1991, 1985 to 1991, and 1984 to 1991 in both non-diabetic and diabetic patients. The same reference groups were used as in the previous analysis, but a censored model at 1984 was used for the formaldehyde patients. This was done to compare as closely as possible the impact of the entry year. Only age, renal diagnosis, diabetes, and co-morbidity were evaluated. Figure 10 shows the effect of the entry year working back from 1988. At no point was a P-value of less than 0.05 achieved, yet there was a change in the direction of the peracetic acid effect from less than one relative risk of death in the 1988 to 1991 patients to greater than one as patients from earlier years were entered in both non-diabetic and diabetic patient groups for analysis.

To evaluate further the above findings of an increasing effect of the 1984 switch year, we calculated the mean Kt/V for non-diabetic and diabetic patient cohorts for the years 1976 to 1982, 1983, 1984, 1985, 1986, 1987, 1988, and

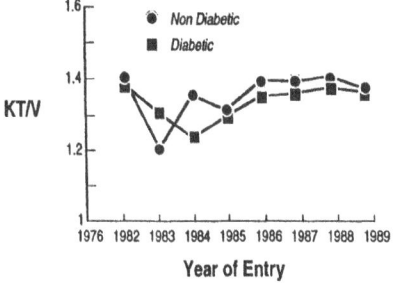

Fig. 11. The mean Kt/V of cohorts of patients entering each year after 1976 to 1982. The Kt/V of patients who entered from 1983 to 1985 were lower in both non-diabetic and diabetic patients.

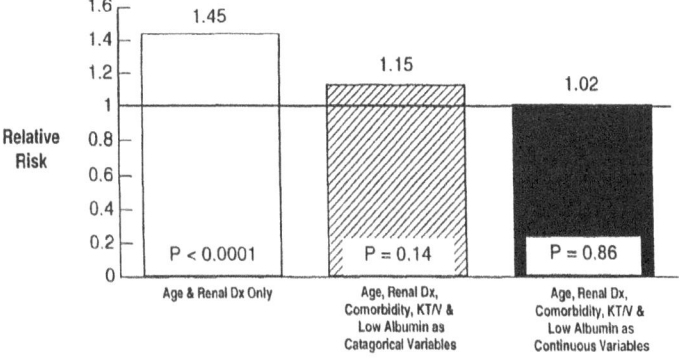

Fig. 12. Comparison of adding confounding variables to the time-dependent Cox regression analysis for peracetic acid relative risk with stratification of non-diabetic and diabetic patients. This shows as co-morbidity, Kt/V, and albumin are added, peracetic acid as a risk factor becomes non-significant.

1989, as shown in Fig. 11. The Kt/Vs delivered to the cohort of patients entering in 1983 to 1985 were less than the patients in earlier and later years. The difference in therapy would have an impact on survival as well as the association of Kt/V with a low serum albumin [25,26]. The analysis was then performed to include Kt/V and albumin as continuous variables compared to an analysis with only age and renal diagnosis without adjustments for the seven co-morbid clinical diseases. Figure 12 shows the time-dependent analysis with age and renal diagnosis only having an adverse effect of peracetic acid with a relative risk of 1.45 (P = < 0.0001). However, when the analysis is performed with all relevant survival factors, including the seven co-morbid risk factors, Kt/V, and albumin as continuous variables and stratified by non-diabetics and diabetics, the effect of peracetic acid reuse in the time-dependent analysis becomes non-significant with a relative risk of 1.02 (P = 0.86), which is equal to formaldehyde as the baseline. These results would reflect a fully adjusted analysis of all the known major risk factors in a time-dependent model.

Discussion

The comparison of hemodialysis patient survival between countries poses a number of problems in interpreting these studies, especially if reuse as a practice is being analyzed as a risk factor. Acceptance rates are significantly higher in the United States, suggesting US patients are entering with increased complexity [27]. We and others have shown that co-morbidity plays a significant role in patient survival, and the complexity of patients is increasing since 1982 [4,13,28]. In addition, Kt/V and a low serum albumin are potent risk factors with each accounting for 30% to 40% of the difference in survival of dialysis patients which adds more complexity to any analysis [28,29,30,31]. The evaluation of Kt/V as a risk factor in patient outcome may be particularly relevant in the United States since inadequate therapy appears to be delivered compared to Europe [4]. Given the noted complexities relative to risk factors of co-morbidity, Kt/V, and a low serum albumin, if unanalyzed, will confound any outcome analysis, since these factors would need to be assumed to be equally distributed in all subgroups.

The same factors mentioned above are equally problematic when evaluating reuse as a risk factor within the United States. Unfortunately, national studies lack the detailed risk factors, which may lead to potential selection bias, complicating the analysis. For example, in the US HCFA reuse study, there was no detail on clinical co-morbidity, Kt/V, or albumin available for the analysis. Without these factors, the study would need to assume, as mentioned above, equal distribution of the important patient and therapy risk factors in the no reuse, formaldehyde, peracetic acid, and glutaraldehyde reuse groups. Unfortunately, no data was presented to validate these assumptions, including the assumption to use free-standing dialysis units only. Therefore, the associations noted in the HCFA study are difficult to interpret, since three major areas of confounding risk factors were not available for analysis.

The study we have performed attempted to determine whether peracetic acid exposure had an effect on survival of hemodialysis patients compared to formaldehyde while analyzing all known risk factors. Since our study covered a long interval and many patients survived through the switching of reuse agents, we chose to use a time-dependent Cox analysis to fully credit all formaldehyde survival time to the formaldehyde era and all peracetic acid survival to the peracetic acid era. In this manner, any potential for biasing the data would be reduced, since no censoring of patients would occur at the switch, and the switch would not be ignored as would be the case in an intent to treat analysis. With the time-dependent approach, we did not find a significant effect of peracetic acid reuse or exposure on patient survival when only age, renal diagnosis, and the seven co-morbid risk factors were entered into the model. The direction of the non-significant effect, however, was still greater than 1.0 compared to formaldehyde and was further evaluated with additional detail to be sure the effect was not a result of an insufficient sample size.

We further analyzed the year of entry as a factor to determine if cohorts of patients entering after 1982 had any therapy index (Kt/V) confounding effects. The demographics of the Kt/V cohorts by entry year clearly showed lower values between the 1983 to 1985 interval, which would require adjustments in the Cox analysis. Since we had previously shown a low albumin was associated with a Kt/V $\leq$ 1.2 in non-diabetics [25,26], this meant that adjustments for a low albumin would also be required as well as the fact that albumin is a strong independent risk factor in all patients. The magnitude of the relative risk of death associated with peracetic acid was markedly reduced to 1.02 (P-value of 0.86) compared to formaldehyde showing the analysis was altered considerably by the added detail of co-morbidity, Kt/V, and albumin as continuous variables. Therefore, within our own dialysis program, given the details of water treatment, control of microbiology, and the maintenance of dialyzer clearance with reuse, we do not find peracetic acid reuse to be a risk factor for survival of hemodialysis patients compared to formaldehyde.

Reflecting back on the HCFA national reuse study, it is difficult to interpret the statistical association with increased risks associated with germicides. Unfortunately, sufficient detail was not available in the HCFA study to evaluate co-morbidity, Kt/V, or albumin. In addition, although not analyzed here, no data was available on the impact of hematocrit on patient outcome, since erythropoietin was introduced in July of 1989, which would potentially be another confounding variable. Our own data has shown an impact of a lower risk of death when the hematocrit was greater than 29% hematocrit (mean 32%) compared to under 29% (mean 26%) [32]. These factors, as well as the others presented in our study, demonstrated the complexity of this issue and the detail required in a retrospective epidemiologic analysis of dialysis patient outcome. Further studies on a larger sample size from more dialysis providers will be required, but these analyses should include all known risk factors to eliminate any potential study biases and confounding variables with known effects.

Summary

Survival of hemodialysis patients is influenced by many factors including age, hypertension, renovascular disease, diabetes, clinical co-morbidity, delivered dialysis reflected by the Kt/V, and low serum albumin. Reuse practices as a risk factor has not previously been evaluated with adjustments for the above factors. We studied 1773 hemodialysis patients from 1976 to 1989 for the effect of peracetic acid reuse compared to formaldehyde reuse in a time-dependent Cox regression analysis adjusting for age, renal diagnosis, seven clinical co-morbid conditions, Kt/V, and low serum albumin. The results show if only age and renal diagnosis are evaluated, peracetic acid reuse was associated with an increased relative risk of death of 47% compared to formaldehyde reuse. However, after adjusting for the additional factors of co-morbidity, Kt/V, and a low albumin, the relative risk for peracetic acid was reduced to 1.02 with a P-value of 0.86. We conclude if confounding variables such as co-morbidity, Kt/V, and serum albumin are not taken into consideration, peracetic acid reuse is associated with an increased risk of death. However, when all risks are evaluated, peracetic acid was not a risk factor in our dialysis program.

Acknowledgments

The authors wish to extend their sincere appreciation to Dr. Chap Le of the University of Minnesota Biostatistics Department for long-standing consultation. In addition, the authors acknowledge the countless hours the RKDP Information Services staff devoted to data collection over the past 18 years, as well as the assistance in manuscript preparation by Dana Knopic and Diane Erickson.

References

1. Tokars JI, Alter MJ, Favero MS. National surveillance of dialysis-associated diseases in the United States, 1991. US Department of Health and Human Services, Centers for Disease Control, Atlanta, Georgia, 1991
2. Medicare Program. Standards for the reuse of hemodialyzer filters and other dialysis supplies. 42 Code of Federal Regulations, Part 405, October 2, 1987
3. Association for the Advancement of Medical Instrumentation. AAMI recommended practice for hemodialyzers. Washington DC, June 1993
4. US Renal Data System. USRDS 1992 Annual Data Report, The National Institutes of Health, National Institute of Diabetes and Digestive and Kidney Diseases, Bethesda, Maryland, August 1991
5. US Renal Data System. USRDS 1991 Annual Data Report, The National Institutes of Health, National Institute of Diabetes and Digestive and Kidney Diseases, Bethesda, Maryland, August 1990
6. US Renal Data System. USRDS 1990 Annual Data Report, The National Institutes of Health, National Institute of Diabetes and Digestive and Kidney Diseases, Bethesda, Maryland, August 1989
7. US Renal Data System. USRDS 1989 Annual Data Report, The National Institutes of Health, National Institute of Diabetes and Digestive and Kidney Diseases, Bethesda, Maryland, August 1988
8. Eggers P. Mortality rates among dialysis patients in medicare's end-stage renal disease program. Am J Kidney Dis 1990; 15(5): 414–421.
9. Disney A. Prescription and practice of dialysis in Australia, 1988. Am J Kidney Dis 1990; 15(5): 494–499.
10. Disney A. Dialysis treatment in Australia, 1982 to 1988. Am J Kidney Dis 1990; 15(5): 402–409.
11. Held P, Brunner F, Odaka M, Garcia J, Port F, Gaylin D. Five-year survival for end-stage renal disease patients in the United States, Europe, and Japan, 1982 to 1987. Am J Kidney Dis 1990; 15(5): 451–457.
12. Gotch F, Yarian S, Keen M. A kinetic survey of US hemodialysis prescriptions. Am J Kidney Dis 1990; 15(5): 511–515.

13. Collins A, Hanson G, Umen A, Kjellstrand C, Keshaviah P. Changing risk factor demographics in end-stage renal disease patients entering hemodialysis and the impact on long-term mortality. Am J Kidney Dis 1990; 15(5): 422–432.

14. Kjellstrand C, Hylander B, Collins A. Mortality on dialysis – on the influence of early start, patient characteristics, and transplantation and acceptance rates. Am J Kidney Dis 1990; 15(5): 483–490.

15. Shaldon S, Koch K. Survival and adequacy in long-term hemodialysis. Nephron 1991; 59: 353–357.

16. Shaldon S. Adequacy of long-term hemodialysis. Current Opinion in Nephrology and Hypertension 1992; 1: 197–202.

17. Benson J. New studies on dialyzer germicides. (Letter to hemodialysis personnel) Department of Health and Human Services, Public Health Service, Food and Drug Administration, Rockville, Maryland, October 26, 1992.

18. Berkseth R, Luehmann D, Mcmichael C, Keshaviah P, Kjellstrand C. Peracetic acid for reuse of hemodialyzers clinical studies. Trans Am Soc Artif Intern Organs 1984; 30: 270–275.

19. Hume R, Weyers E. Relationship between total body water and surface area in normal and obese subjects. J Clin Pathol 1971; 24: 234–238.

20. Umen AJ, Le C. Prognostic factors, models and related statistical problems in the survival of end-stage renal disease patients on hemodialysis. Stat Med 1986; 5: 637–652.

21. Collins A, Keshaviah P, Berkseth R, Ilstrup K, Mcmichael C, Ebben J. Short efficient hemodialysis with reduced symptoms. Kidney Int 1984; 27: 158.

22. Keshaviah P, Luehmann D, Ilstrup K, Collins A. Technical requirements for rapid high-efficiency therapy. Artificial Organs 1986; 10(3): 189–194.

23. Keshaviah P, Berkseth R, Ilstrup K, Mcmichael C, Collins A. Reduced treatment time: hemodialysis (HD) versus hemofiltration (HF). Trans Am Soc Int Organs 1985; 31: 176–182.

24. Keshaviah P, Collins A. High-efficiency hemodialysis. *In*: GD D'Amico and G Colasanti, editors, Contributions to Nephrology, Volume 69, S Karger, Publisher, 109–119, 1989

25. Collins A, Keshaviah P, Ma J, Umen A. How important is serum albumin as a predictor of mortality? (abstract). Am Soc Artif Int Org 1992; 21: 82.

26. Collins A, Keshaviah P, Ma J, Umen A. Infectious death rate is increased with a low serum albumin $\leq$ 3.5 gm/dl. (abstract). Am Soc Nephr 1992; 3(3): 360.

27. Health Care Financing Research Report. End Stage Renal Disease, 1991. Department of Health and Human Services, Health Care Financing Administration, Bureau of Data Management and Strategy, Office of Research and Demonstrations, Baltimore, Maryland, May 1993

28. Collins A, Ma J, Umen A, Keshaviah P. Urea index (Kt/V) and other predictors of hemodialysis patient survival. Am J Kidney Dis (submitted)

29. Lowrie E, Lew N. Death risk in hemodialysis patients: the predictive value of commonly measured variables and an evaluation of death rate differences between facilities. Am J Kidney Dis 1990; 15(5): 458–482.

30. Collins A, Liao M, Umen A, Hanson G, Keshaviah P. Diabetic hemodialysis patients treated with a high Kt/V have a lower risk of death than standard Kt/V. (abstract). J Am Soc Nephr 1991; 2(3): 318.

31. Collins A, Liao M, Umen A, Hanson G, Keshaviah P. High-efficiency bicarbonate hemodialysis has a lower risk of death than standard acetate dialysis. (abstract). J Am Soc Nephr 1991; 2(3): 318.

32. Collins A, Ma J, Umen A. Infectious and all-cause death rates in hemodialysis patients are lower with a mean hematocrit of 32% versus 26%. (abstract). International Congress of Nephrology, June, 1993.

CHAPTER 8

Twenty-five years of safe reuse

CHRISTOPHER R. BLAGG, TOM K. SAWYER and GREG BISCHAK

Dialyzer reuse and its potential relationship to mortality is a subject which recurrently attracts attention and strongly held views. This paper traces the history of dialyzer reuse as practiced over the years at the Northwest Kidney Centers in Seattle, Washington, and comments on some of the issues which undoubtedly will be discussed in detail by others.

In 1964, Shaldon and coworkers in England described a process in which coil dialyzers were refrigerated after use, storing the dialyzer and its contained anticoagulated blood between dialyses [1]. While often described as dialyzer reuse, this technique did not involve cleaning and resterilization of the dialyzer and so perhaps might better be described as interrupted dialysis.

At that time the Kiil flat plate dialyzer was being used for maintenance hemodialysis in Seattle, and so attempts at reuse were made with refrigeration of the dialyzer using citrate as anticoagulant. Pyrogen reactions were frequent, the technique was cumbersome, the refrigerator storage was difficult, and so this approach was soon dropped.

Prior to 1973

Between 1965 and 1967, the Division of Nephrology at the University of Washington was developing techniques to improve the return of blood to the patient from the Kiil dialyzer at the end of dialysis. This included studies of air rinse and saline rinse procedures, and led to the development of a tilt cart for the Kiil dialyzer to facilitate blood return. As these techniques were refined, it became possible to return almost all the residual blood to the patient. This facilitated dialyzer cleaning and made reuse possible without refrigeration [2].

The original motivation for developing a dialyzer reuse technique was to reduce both the cost of dialysis in the home and the effort required of patient and family in disassembling, rebuilding, leak testing and sterilizing the 65-pound Kiil dialyzer before every dialysis. By 1967, almost all dialysis patients in Seattle were performing hemodialysis overnight for twelve hours three times weekly at home using a Kiil dialyzer and most were also working full time. Once assembled, the Kiil dialyzer was subject to an appreciable

E. A. Friedman (ed.), Death on Hemodialysis, 83–90.
© 1994 Kluwer Academic Publishers.

frequency of leakage when air tested prior to sterilization. If leakage occurred, the dialyzer had to be disassembled and rebuilt. Reuse reduced the need for patients to rebuild their dialyzers as frequently, and they were trained to use their dialyzer for three to six dialyses before rebuilding. The dialyzer could then be disassembled, cleaned and rebuilt at the weekend when there would be less interference with workday demands.

Criteria for the cleaning agent were: (1) ability to remove blood, fibrin, and white cell deposits from the cellophane membrane and polyvinyl tubing surfaces; (2) effective cleaning without damaging the membranes or other components of the dialyzer; (3) capability to detect residual amounts by a simple test; (4) a chemically pure, relatively non-toxic substance that is easily removed from the dialyzer and which will ensure safety to the patient despite long-term exposure to trace amounts; and (5) low cost. After investigating several agents, the one selected was a dilute solution of sodium hypochlorite at a temperature of 120° to 160°F and a pH of 11.0. Hypochlorite solution tended to weaken the cellophane membrane by attacking its organic bonds, but use of 15 ml of 14.5% sodium hypochlorite per liter of tap water (1,000 ppm of available chlorine) allowed adequate cleaning without excessive weakening of the membranes.

The technique developed involved tilting the dialyzer and returning as much blood as possible to the patient, draining fluid from the dialysate compartment, and filling the blood circuit with sodium hypochlorite solution while pressurizing the blood compartment to not more than 200 mm, Hg. After a maximum exposure time of 15 minutes the blood compartment was flushed with cold tap water at 1.5 L/min for 10 minutes, and the blood circuit, blood tubing, and dialysate compartment were filled with 1.5% formaldehyde (4% Formalin) for resterilization and storage. Prior to use, the blood circuit was rinsed with 100 ml of heparinized normal saline, and the blood compartment was dialyzed against tap water or dextrose-free dialysate at 500 ml/min for 30 minutes. The blood compartment was then further rinsed with the remaining 900 ml of heparinized normal saline and the rinse fluid tested for residual formaldehyde by Clinitest.

Because the blood tubing sets could be sterilized and reused at the same time, it was estimated the annual saving could be as much as $700 per year per patient. As the cost of home dialysis at that time was between $4,000 and $5,000 a year (excluding the cost of the fluid supply system), this saving was significant. The money generated was used to provide treatment for needy patients.

The 1967 initial report [2] noted that no untoward patient reactions had occurred and that cultures of the blood circuit had been uniformly sterile. Patients' BUN levels and creatinine clearances did not change significantly with reuse. Nevertheless, after four or five 16-hour dialyses, excessive membrane coating became obvious.

The 1970s to the 1980s

The advent of pre-sterilized, disposable flat plate hemodialyzers from Gambro resolved the problem of convenience but was associated with an increased cost. By 1972 the Northwest Kidney Center was treating all patients who were referred, irrespective of ability to pay. Thus, the only way to introduce these new, efficient and convenient dialyzers was to use them more than once. To accomplish this, the Kiil dialyzer reuse technique was modified so that it was possible to meet a goal of six uses per dialyzer. The technique used was similar to that described independently some years later by others [3]. With six uses the cost of a two year supply of disposable dialyzers was roughly equivalent to the cost of a non-disposable dialyzer.

With the start of the Medicare End Stage Renal Disease Program in 1973, cost saving ceased to be an important consideration for patients dialyzing as outpatients because of the initial relatively generous reimbursement for this treatment modality by Medicare and the low cost of the disposable dialyzers available at that time. For the next ten years the Northwest Kidney Center used both flat plate and hollow fiber dialyzers for outpatient dialysis without reuse.

In contrast, home hemodialysis was poorly reimbursed until passage of the Medicare Amendments of 1978. Consequently, the policy of the Northwest Kidney Center was to encourage reuse of disposable dialyzers in the home for all non-diabetic patients. Dialyzer reuse was usually not recommended for the few diabetic patients treated at that time as their heparin dosage was usually minimized to reduce the risk of retinal hemorrhage. During home hemodialysis training, patients were taught to reuse. Their dialyzers were examined to establish they could be reused effectively and they were trained to use a flat plate dialyzer three to six times and a hollow fiber dialyzer three times. Emphasis was on a simple manual procedure, careful training and testing, discussion of the risks associated with failure to follow procedures precisely, adherence to a check list, and the importance of documentation.

The technique used was essentially similar for both hollow fiber and flat plate dialyzers except that following an initial water rinse, with flat plate dialyzers bleach solution was used to clean the blood compartment, while with hollow fiber dialyzers a fiber bundle routine volume measurement was made. With both types of dialyzers, blood and dialysate compartments were sterilized and stored with formaldehyde, and a saline rinse was used prior to dialysis together with a Clinitest to check for formaldehyde removal.

At the time this experience was reported in 1983 [5], the Northwest Kidney Center had 226 home hemodialysis patients of whom 140 (62%) reused their dialyzers. A questionnaire was used to gather information from all home dialysis patients about dialyzer reuse and their attitudes to this. Sixty percent of patients responded to the questionnaire, of whom 73 percent reused their dialyzers. Seventy five percent of 101 patients using flat plate dialyzers reused, averaging 4.3 uses per dialyzer. Blood leaks were reported as frequent by 4 percent of patients, but more than one-third had never had a blood leak. One-third of patients had never noticed fibrin build-up, but 20 percent noted this as a frequent occurrence. Eighty-six percent of the patients had never had an episode of fever. Thirty-seven patients used hollow fiber dialyzers, and 24 (65 percent) of them reused for an average of 3 uses. The frequency of blood leaks was less than with flat plate dialyzers. Fibrin build up was also noted less frequently, although this probably represented selection because patients known to have fibrin problems were more likely to be trained to use a flat plate dialyzer. Eighty percent of these patients had not had an episode of fever.

At the time of survey, the duration of home hemodialysis in the patients reusing their dialyzers averaged 3 years and 11 months, and the patients represented more than 500 patient years of experience.

For 46 percent of the patients, reuse was done by the family member or live-in friend who assisted the patient with hemodialysis, and 35 percent did the reuse procedure themselves. A paid dialysis helper carried out reuse for the remaining 24 percent of patients.

In patients who responded to the survey, the commonest reason for not reusing their dialyzers was because of physician or staff advice, usually related to problems with fibrin formation. Another common reason for not doing reuse at home was the time taken and the patient's post-dialysis fatigue. Four patients reported problems with formaldehyde sensitivity, three were worried about the potential risk of infection and blood leaks, and three were concerned because the manufacturer's label said the dialyzer was for one time use only.

The conclusion, based of 14 years experience, was that dialyzer reuse by properly trained home hemodialysis patients was a safe procedure, and there had been "no major patient problems resulting from this practice". Dialyzer reuse in the home was estimated to save some $3,200 annually for each patient reusing. Again, the savings were used to help cover the costs of home dialysis helpers for patients without family members, provide housing for out-of-town patients while they received home dialysis training, pay for transportation for home dialysis patients from remote areas who needed backup dialysis or other services, support periodic home visits by the training staff, pay for medications for needy patients, provide increased social work staff, and pay for numerous individual social support situations [4].

1983 to 1993

The last ten years have seen further changes in dialyzer reuse at the Northwest Kidney Centers.

First, home hemodialysis patients are no longer expected to reuse unless they are on high flux dialysis. Once again, the main reason for this change was the time and effort required for reuse at the end of dialysis. Rather, most home hemodialysis patients use standard hollow fiber or flat plate dialyzers one time only.

In contrast, patients on outpatient hemodialysis are now routinely expected to reuse dialyzers, although this is not compulsory. This policy was introduced as a result of the reduction in Medicare reimbursement with the introduction of the composite rate in 1983. Reuse is mandatory only for patients treated with high flux or other expensive dialyzers. In our experience, with adequate explanation of the issues and risks involved, more than 85 percent of patients are willing to undertake dialyzer reuse. This is performed using semi automated and automated equipment, and the only sterilant we have used is formaldehyde. Currently we use 1.5 percent formaldehyde at 40° C for 24 hours, based on the studies of formaldehyde kinetics by Hakim and coworkers [6]. Again, no major problems have been noted in association with dialyzer reuse. The emphasis in our reuse program always has been on safety rather than on maximizing the number of uses. This, together with careful documentation and monitoring, has contributed to our comfort with dialyzer reuse. Dialyzer reuse and dialysis are safe procedures but are not risk free, being as safe as the technique used and the people doing this, just like any manufacturing process.

In order to address the issue of mortality, we examined the mortality for hemodialysis patients in the Northwest Kidney Centers system over the four years 1988 through 1991 using the method of Wolfe and coworkers [7]. This allows comparison of survival in a patient population with survival data from the US Renal Data System adjusted for age, race and diagnosis. Over these 4 years, 301 deaths would have been expected in the NKC patient population based on national data, but only 257 deaths occurred. The standardized mortality ratio (SMR) by year ranged from 0.76 to 0.91, and the overall mean SMR was 0.85. These results are statistically significantly better than the mortality expected (Chi square = 6.4; $p = 0.05$–0.01). Thus, we see no evidence of an increase in mortality in our patients that can be related to dialyzer reuse.

Obviously, the weakness in this statement is that dialysis patient mortality depends on many factors, and it is impossible for us to say whether or not our patients' survival would have been even better if they had not been exposed to reused dialyzers. We are reexamining our data base to see if there is a significant difference between those treated with reused dialyzers and those who were not.

Discussion

The recent reports to the Food and Drug Administration, based on data from a USRDS case mix study and from the Centers for Disease Control, of an increased relative risk of mortality in patients treated with dialyzers reused with Renalin as sterilant [8] have again precipitated hot debates on the pros and cons of dialyzer reuse [9,10]. The information reported so far, while showing a statistically significant correlation between mortality and dialyzer reuse using Renalin, does not mean that Renalin or dialyzer reuse is the cause of the increased mortality. Many other factors are possibly involved. For example, it has always been our contention and that of others that problems with dialyzer reuse are almost always a manifestation of bad dialysis. This is in keeping with a study by Held and coworkers in 1987 [11]. This study examined five-year survival in 4,661 patients whose first dialysis was in 1977. Apart from the usual correlations they found that the relative risk of death was less (0.88) in dialysis units that had been reusing dialyzers since before 1980. This was statistically significant (p < 0.03). Survival in units which had started dialyzer reuse more recently was unchanged (relative risk = 1.01) and resembled that in patients not treated with reused dialyzers. A likely hypothesis to explain these findings is that the better outcome in long-term reuse units reflected better quality of treatment along dimensions not controlled for in the analysis.

It is also significant that in the recent analysis of mortality and dialyzer reuse the relative risk for patients treated by dialyzers reused with formaldehyde was not statistically different from that in patients who did not reuse dialyzers. This is in keeping with most reports on dialyzer reuse which have not suggested that this is associated with adverse outcomes [12,13,14,15,16].

Nevertheless, the recent reports have restimulated the interest of those who are opposed to dialyzer reuse. These include both physicians [17] and manufacturers and suppliers of dialyzers who clearly would benefit if dialyzer reuse were stopped. However, it is very likely that the increased mortality in US dialysis patients is related to inadequate dialysis as compared with European patients [18]. From the patient's viewpoint, the first concerns should be that they are getting an adequate dose of dialysis delivered, adequate nutrition, and effective control of hypertension.

Where will this lead in the future? First, there must be careful studies to settle once and for all whether dialyzer reuse, when properly carried out, is or is not associated with an increased mortality or other problems in hemodialysis patients. Data which might help should be available from the most recent USRDS case mix study. It is essential this data be analyzed and the results made available as soon as possible. Some of the problems in undertaking studies of the effects of dialyzer reuse are discussed in a critical review of dialyzer reuse by Shusterman and coworkers [19].

If, as we and many others believe, dialyzer reuse, properly carried out, is safe, efforts should be made to develop dialyzers specifically designed to be reused. This should be associated with development of automated equipment which can make the process of reuse more uniform, safe and usable with home hemodialysis. Such equipment should include direct measurement of clearance as a means of ensuring continuing dialyzer efficiency.

Dialyzer reuse currently is relatively uncommon in most western countries and is not practiced at all in Japan. The latter may relate to the fact that Japanese companies produce many of the dialyzers used throughout the world.

Nevertheless, as the cost of health care continues to escalate, there seems no doubt that dialyzer reuse will become the rule everywhere in the future.

However, there is another compelling argument for dialyzer reuse. This relates to the increasing concern for the environment. There are more than 400,000 patients on dialysis throughout the world now. This means that if they all dialyze three times weekly and use a new dialyzer for each dialysis, there are more than 62 million dialyzers, tubing sets, and associated items to be disposed of annually. Disposal of medical waste is already a major and costly item for providers in developed countries, and this will only get worse. Just as the dialysis industry has been a leader in developing sophisticated equipment for dialysis, it is now time for it to lead other health care manufacturers in containing costs and in protecting the environment from its products.

Summary

Dialyzer reuse has been practiced in Seattle for some 25 years without obvious, serious ill effects. We are not convinced that there has been any increased mortality as a result of this, and the complications we have seen have been neither frequent nor serious. We continue to believe that properly done, dialyzer reuse is not only safe but is cost-effective and environmentally beneficial.

Acknowledgements

The authors gratefully acknowledge the efforts of so many staff members of the Northwest Kidney Centers who, over some 25 years, have provided safe dialyzer reuse to so many of our patients. The authors are also indebted to Roberta Leonard for her assistance in preparing this manuscript.

References

1. Shaldon S, Silva H, Rosen S. Technique of refrigerated coil preservation hemodialysis with femoral vein catheterization. Br Med J 1964; 2: 411–413.
2. Pollard TL, Barnett BMS, Eschbach JW, Scribner BH. A technique for the storage and multiple use of the Kiil dialyzer and blood tubing. Trans Amer Soc Artif Int Organs 1967; 3: 24–28.
3. Miach PJ, Evans SM, Wilcox AA, Dawborn JK. Reuse of a disposable dialyzer for home dialysis. Med J Aust 1976; 1: 146–147.
4. Sawyer TK. Dialyzer reuse: home patient considerations. In: Hemodialyzer Reuse: Issues and Solutions. Arlington, VA: Association for the Advancement of Medical Instrumentation, 1985: 64–66.
5. Blagg CR, Pollock P, Wallace J. Home dialysis and dialyzer reuse in Seattle. In: Sadler J, editor. Proceedings of the National Workshop on Reuse of Consumables in Hemodialysis. Washington, DC: Kidney Disease Coalition, 1983, pp 40–47.
6. Hakim RM, Friedrich RA, Lowrie EG with the technical assistance of Mantilla JM, Lee C. Formaldehyde kinetics and bacteriology in dialyzers. Kidney Int 1985; 28: 936–943.
7. Wolfe RA, Gaylin DS, Port FK, Held PJ, Wood CL. Using USRDS generated mortality tables to compare local ESRD mortality rates to national rates. Kidney Int 1992; 42: 991–996.

8. Held PJ, Port FK, Wolfe R, Levin NW, Gaylin D. Oral report, American Society of Nephrology, Baltimore, MD, November 1992.
9. Shaldon S. Reuse. A practice that should be abandoned. Semin Dial 1993; 6: 11–12.
10. Levin NW. Dialyzer reuse: a currently acceptable practice. Semin Dial 1993; 6: 89–90.
11. Held PJ, Pauly MV, Diamond L. Survival analysis of patients undergoing dialysis. JAMA 1987; 257: 645–650.
12. Bok DV, Pascaul L, Herberger C, Sawyer R, Levin NW. Effect of multiple use of dialyzers on intradialytic symptoms. Proc Clin Dial Transplant Forum 1980; 10: 92–99.
13. Wineman RJ. New technologies in automated reprocessing of hemodialyzers. Assoc Advance Med Instr Tech Anal Rev, 1985, pp 50–55.
14. Kant K, Pollak V, Cathey M, Goetz D, Berlin R. Multiple use of dialyzers; safety and efficiency. Kidney Int 1984; 19: 728–738.
15. Pollak VE, Kant SK, Parnell SL, Levin NW. Repeated use of dialyzers is safe; long-term observations on morbidity and mortality in patients with end-stage renal disease. Nephron 1986; 42: 217–223.
16. Wing AJ, Brunner HOA, Chantler C. Mortality and morbidity of reusing dialyzers. Br Med J 1978; 2: 853–855.
17. Shaldon S, Koch KM. Survival and adequacy in long-term hemodialysis. Nephron 1991; 59: 353–357.
18. Held PJ, Blagg CR, Liska DW, Port FK, Hakim R, Levin N. The dose of hemodialysis according to dialysis prescription in Europe and the United States. Kidney Int 1992; 42 (Suppl 38): S16–S21.
19. Shusterman NH, Feldman HI, Wasserstein A, Strom BL. Reprocessing of hemodialyzers: a critical appraisal. Amer J Kidney Dis 1989; 14: 81–89.

CHAPTER 9

Reuse accelerates death

JOHN D. BOWER

"Reprocessing of dialyzers when practiced following federally approved policies and procedures is both safe and efficacious"; so states the policy of the Renal Physicians Association. The American Association of Kidney Patients "recognizes that treatment for end stage renal disease is a dynamic evolving process where continued improvements are occurring. Medical benefits of reprocessing dialyzers for the majority of patients have not been clearly defined through replicable blinded statistically significant studies." [1] In spite of this apparent difference of opinion in the policy statement on reprocessing of hemodialyzers that was issued jointly by the American Association of Kidney Patients and the Renal Physicians Association, the practice of reuse continues to expand, and indeed the majority of patients being treated with hemodialysis are being treated with reprocessed dialyzers.

The recent national release of data by the United States Renal Data System (USRDS), National Institutes of Health (NIH), Communicable Disease Control and Prevention (CDC&P) and the Food and Drug Administration (FDA) showing an increased mortality associated with reuse, particularly with certain sterilizing agents, suggests that the practice of reuse may not be as safe and as efficacious as once thought. Maybe short term studies by isolated dialysis facilities with economic interests in reuse cannot reflect the big picture. There are many other examples in our society where it has taken extensive research over many years to establish a cause and effect relationship. Cigarette smoking and the use of all tobacco products is just one example of a delayed cause and effect observation. The devastating injury inflicted on our patients by the use of aluminum containing compounds to control phosphorus in end stage renal disease patients is another. We now know that after 20 years of aluminum binders that indeed they do produce a serious bone disease and also produce a fatal syndrome called dialysis dementia. It took a long time to demonstrate a cause and effect relationship for cigarettes and aluminum. How can we assume that reuse is O.K. when roughly 25% of our patients die each year? What we do know is that reuse is cost effective and economically efficacious for the provider.

E. A. Friedman (ed.), Death on Hemodialysis, 91–94.

The predominant driving force for reuse of disposable dialyzers is exclusively economic. The First Use Syndrome has been used as a 'straw man'. The FDA incident reports show First Use Syndrome occurs very rarely compared to numerous pyrogenic reactions associated with reuse. It is doubtful that the First Use Syndrome even occurs at all, but there is little doubt about the pyrogenicity of the improperly reprocessed dialyzer [2]. It is also difficult to ignore the 13 deaths in a single unit where improper reprocessing of dialyzers was associated with a Mycobacterium chelonei outbreak. These data suggest that all may not be well with reuse, in spite of the fact that the majority of patients in the US are being treated with reprocessed dialyzers. The numerous reactions to pyrogen and the deaths from septicemia provide direct evidence that a breakdown in the reuse process can and does occur.

There is also good indirect evidence that reuse of dialyzers accelerates death. When the National Dialysis Cooperative Study was performed, a minimal gold standard for dialysis was established in the mind of the practicing nephrologist [3,4]. This was expressed in the formulation of Kt/V and a solid sacred number was presented and readily accepted by the nephrological community as adequate dialysis. Once this formula was presented, the nephrologists could quite readily establish the time (t) that the patient should be dialyzed and then began a search for a dialyzer that would give them the coefficient (K) to permit this shortened dialysis. The price of these high efficient or high flux dialyzers was close to prohibitive if they were not going to be reprocessed. As a result, the reuse of expensive dialyzers indirectly fostered short time dialysis with a further increase in our mortality. The urgent need to do dialysis for less than three hours was necessary in order to permit a dialysis facility that was staffed for 10 hours a day to perform three dialysis treatments during a single shift. The practice of reuse in association with shortened dialysis time brought about tremendous savings both in labor and in consumable supplies. The increased mortality associated with these practices is well known [5,6,7].

Another indirect effect of reuse to increase mortality resulted from short dialysis and the failure to control blood pressure. It has been suggested in several studies that shorter dialysis does not permit optimal control of volume, thereby leading to hypertension [8]. When the blood pressure is not controlled or requires multiple medications to control it, the mortality rate will increase. Reprocessed dialyzers do not maintain the same ultrafiltration capacity. This can cause sporadic and unpredictable fluid removal and lead to hypertension.

One argument supporting reuse is enhanced biocompatability of the reprocessed membranes. Many studies have been carried out demonstrating that activation of the complement system does occur – particularly associated with cellulosic membranes. This observation implies that this is bad for the patient. This has not been shown to be the case in clinical trials. It has been reported that this 'biocompatability' is improved with reuse. The persons practicing reuse have not looked at the membranes for residual debris. When the membranes of a dialyzer to be reprocessed are stained immunologically, it has been demonstrated that these membranes are heavily coated with IgA, IgG, IgM, fibrinogen, albumin, C3, and beta 2 microglobulin.

Specific staining for these blood components demonstrates extensive adherence to the membrane. These membranes are then subjected to treatment with heat, formaldehyde or other sterilizing agents which invoke their bacteriocidal consequence by denaturing protein. Tremendous quantities of denatured protein are then infused back into, hopefully, the same patient with each subsequent dialysis on a reprocessed dialyzer. The long range impact of this massive infusion of denatured protein has yet to be investigated. In view of the fact that the overwhelming majority of our patients are dying of some form of idiopathic cardiomyopathy, it may be worthwhile to investigate the possible cause and effect relationship between the practice of reprocessing dialyzers and the increased death rate from cardiomyopathy.

In a single dialysis chain which has over 1,000 patients, reuse of dialyzers has never been practiced. The gross mortality rate in this dialysis chain has been less than 17% for the years of 1990 (.16), 1991 (.15), and 1992 (.17). Using the Wolfe model to calculate the SMR, the mortality rate has been 0.68, 0.80, and 0.79 for the years 1990, 1991, and 1992 respectively. When the gross mortality rate of this single dialysis chain is compared to the other facilities in the state who use reprocessed dialyzers, the gross mortality rate is 17% as compared to 25%. Comparing the mortality rate of the nonreuse facilities in the three state Network to the facilities that practice reuse, there is a 7% difference in gross mortality. These gross mortality relationships are not changed when the SMR is calculated using the Wolfe formula. These data basically mirror image the data that was presented by HCFA comparing reuse to nonreuse. Mortality is increased in facilities that reprocess dialyzers regardless of the sterilant used.

In conclusion, there is direct as well as indirect evidence that reuse of dialyzers accelerates death. (1) The direct evidence is the increased incidence of pyrogen reactions and mortality associated with infection. (2) It is very apparent that not all reuse is done properly all of the time by all of the facilities. (3) The indirect evidence is that there is an increased mortality associated with shorter dialysis and difficulties with blood pressure control as a result of the reuse of expensive high flux, high efficiency dialyzers. (4) There are a large number of blood components that are left adhering to any reprocessed membrane. These blood products and cell fragments are then denatured and infused back into the patient. (5) The US has the highest mortality rate of any developed nation in the world as far as hemodialysis is concerned. The US is also the only nation that reuses disposable dialyzers in the majority of its ESRD population. (6) The recent data presented by several federal agencies suggest that reuse is not as safe as nonreuse. (7) It could only be concluded that reuse should be discontinued until such time as it can be conclusively demonstrated that it is a safe and effective procedure when performed properly and that it does not accelerate death.

References

1. American Association of Kidney Patients; Renal Physicians Association. Policy Statement on Reprocessing of Hemodialyzers. July 1987.
2. Gordon SM, Tipple M, Bland LA, Jarvis WR. Pyrogenic reactions associated with the reuse of disposable hollow-fiber hemodialyzers. JAMA 1988; 260: 2077–2081.
3. Laird NM, Berkey CS, Lowrie EG. Modeling success or failure of dialysis therapy: The National Cooperative Dialysis Study. Kidney Int 1983; 23(Supp 13): S101–S106.
4. Gotch FA, Sargent JA. A mechanistic analysis of the National Cooperative Dialysis Study. Kidney Int 1985; 28: 526–534.
5. Held PJ, Levin NW, Bovbjerg RR, Pauly MV. Mortality and duration of hemodialysis treatment. JAMA 1991; 265: 871–875.
6. Berger EE, Lowrie EG. Mortality and the length of dialysis. JAMA 1991; 265: 909–910.
7. Wizemann V, Kramer W. Short-term dialysis – Long-term complications; Ten years experience with short-duration renal replacement therapy. Blood Purifications 1987; 5: 193–201.
8. Charra B, Calemard E, Ruffet M, Chazot C. Survival as an index of adequacy of dialysis. Kidney Int 1992; 41: 1286–1291.

CHAPTER 10

Reuse kills and everyone knows so

STANLEY SHALDON

Introduction

Three decades after the introduction of maintenance hemodialysis as a successful replacement therapy for end stage renal disease, the nephrology world is still preoccupied by a fundamental question; namely how much dialysis therapy is adequate? The recent publication in the US of comparative statistical data suggesting that end stage renal disease patients in Europe and Japan have a significantly better chance of survival than do their counterparts in the US [1] has stimulated me to look closely at differences in the way dialysis is administered in the three major industrialised areas of the world.

A recent editorial review highlighted these differences [2] which are represented graphically in Fig. 1 and may be summarised as follows:
 (1) There are clear differences in gross mortality rates between America on the one hand and Europe and Japan on the other hand.
 (2) The percentage of short hour treatment as defined as less than 10.5 hrs per week is significantly higher in the US.
 (3) The practice of reuse of dialysers is very extensive in the US (> 70%), nonexistent in Japan and negligible in Europe (< 10%).
The purpose of this article will to be to examine the facts available regarding reuse of dialysers and whether this practice could contribute to the higher mortality rates seen in the US.

Nobody used to discuss reuse, and yet the reuse of dialysers has been increasing rapidly in America. Between 1976 and 1989 the number of centers reusing in the US increased from 18% (135 centres) to 68% (1172 centres). The number of patients reusing increased from 6079 (18%) to 89322 (73%) in the same time period [3]. In contrast, the incidence of reuse in Europe is only 10% [4] and in Japan reuse is not practised. Therefore, it seemed reasonable to discuss whether reuse could play a role in the increasing mortality rates recently reported from the US [1]. This now seems even more reasonable since a recent study showed a significant increase in relative mortality risks (1.12 (reuse) (v) 1.0 single use) for over 66,000 patients on hemodialysis in the US during 1989–1990. This means that for every 100 patient deaths with

95

E. A. Friedman (ed.), Death on Hemodialysis, 95–100.
© 1994 Kluwer Academic Publishers.

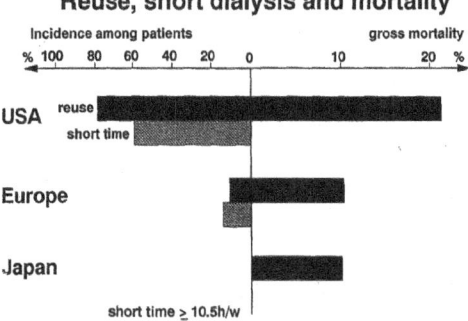

Fig. 1.   The percentage incidence of dialyser reuse, gross mortality and short hour dialysis (defined as less than 10.5hrs per week) in United States, Europe and Japan circa 1988. (Data from Held et al [1], Alter et al [3].

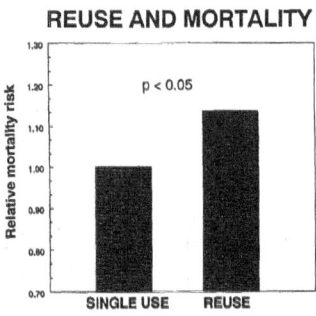

Fig. 2.   The relative risk of dying is significantly higher with reused dialysers than with single use dialysers [5].

single use there were 112 deaths for patients with reused dialysers (Fig. 2) [5]. This more recent observation confirms an earlier one by Held of the doubling of the risk of death in patients dialysed for less than $3\frac{1}{2}$ hours compared to patients dialysed for more than $4\frac{1}{4}$ hours. The incidence of reuse for the individual patient was significantly higher (72.7%) in the short dialysis group than in the long dialysis group (42.9%) [6].

Thus, while the statistical association between reuse and increased mortality now seems clear, the logical explanation for the association of reuse and a higher mortality rate is obviously complex and not immediately evident. Two possibilities occur, the first, that there is an undetected progressive loss of dialyser function which lead to underdialysis. The second is the possibility that reuse increases the bioburden from pyrogen and bacterial contamination of the reprocessed dialyser. This, then leads to an enhanced chronic inflammatory response by the patient.

In the first instance, it is known that there is a loss of surface area of the dialyser usually due to blocking of the individual capillary fibre by thrombus. Methods to measure the loss of fibre bundle volume have been recommended. The most popular method has been to weigh the dialyser before and after an air rinse. The difference in weight will equal the fluid occupying the open capillaries and thus measure the effective surface area remaining after an individual dialysis. It is usually recommended not to reuse the dialyser if the fibre bundle volume loss exceeds 20%. The relation between fibre bundle volume loss and loss of clearance was theoretical and confirmed in only 3 experiments using an HFAK model 3 dialyser (Cordis Dow) in 1974 [7]. It is not surprising that the validity of the loss of fibre bundle volume as a measure of dialyser function in the individual patient has been questioned over the past 17 years. Large series have confirmed the correspondence between fibre loss and clearance [8], but never with point data from the individual patient. Thus, a recent report suggested that there was an excellent preservation of urea clearance which correlated well with fibre bundle volume constancy for up to 14 reuses [9]. However, the data reported was clearly selective and one must assume that the unreported experience (30% of data) implied reuse was abandoned for unexplained reasons. This suggests that the reuse technique was not as predictable as the authors would wish to imply. It is of interest, therefore, that severe dialyser dysfunction with reuse has been reported even though the fibre-bundle volume test was satisfactory. The discrepancy was attributed to preferential channeling of blood and dialysate due to distortion of the fibres by the reuse process [10].

Theoretically, it can be shown that at high blood flows (350 ml/min) as opposed to low blood flows (200 ml/min) there is a loss of clearance with loss of surface area that is not compensated for by an increase in the linear velocity (Fig. 3). This leads to the possibility that reuse up to 20% reduction in fiber bundle volume will lead to significant loss of urea clearance.

A recent report has confirmed this suspicion of progressive loss of urea clearance *in vivo* with reuse. *In vivo*, 1087 urea clearances were measured in over 300 patients and a progressive loss of clearance with reuse of up to 13% was observed. This was not correlated with loss of fibre bundle volume. In addition, initial *in vivo* clearances were at least 10% below *in vitro* data. Thus the theoretical prescription of dialysis by Kt/V would overestimate dialysis dose by more than 20% if reuse was employed [11].

Thus, if one takes into account that there has been a marked increase in blood flow rates with the shortening of dialysis times in the last decade in the US, the loss of clearance occasioned by reuse could clearly contribute to the underdialysis situation in the US today. Indirect evidence that reuse is contributing to underdialysis in America may be gleaned from the less than complete reporting of Sargent who analysed causes for shortfalls in the delivery of dialysis using urea kinetic modeling [12]. Amongst many factors was the dialyser clearance deviation from the manufacturers specification implying less clearance than normal. No mention was made of the role of reuse

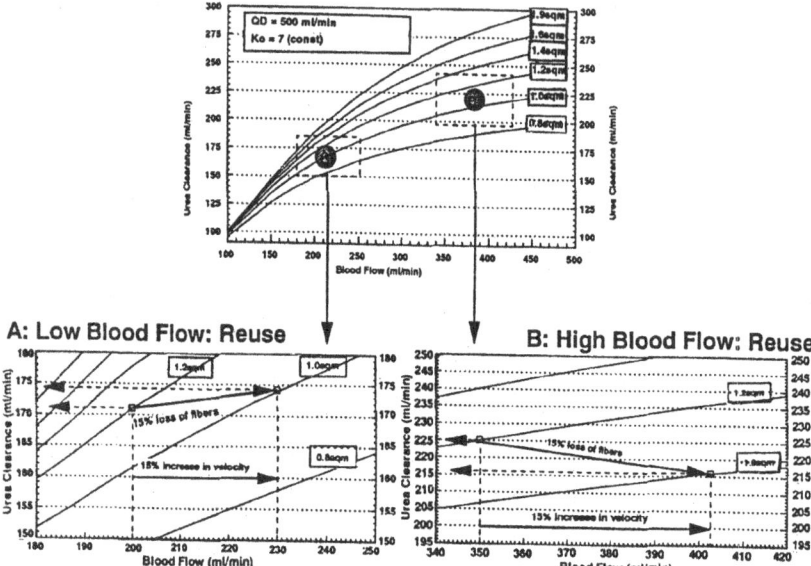

Fig. 3. The influence of surface area and blood flow on urea clearance. K_o = overall mass clearance. Q_d = dialysate flow ml/min. (a) When the blood flow is 200 ml/min, there is actually a small increase in clearance with a loss of 15% of surface area. (b) When the blood flow is 350 ml/min there is a loss of clearance of 5% for a fiber bundle loss of 15%.

in this observation. Clearly, if the analysis was based upon reused dialysers, failure to achieve clearance specifications given by the manufacturer would not be surprising. Similarly, Gotch, in an analysis of transient patients dialysed in his unit from all over the US [13], concluded that inadequate prescription of dialysis based upon urea kinetic modeling was very frequent in the US. Again he did not discuss the variable role of loss of clearance associated with reuse in his analysis. One must assume that in light of the recently presented reuse and mortality data, such hiatuses in the review literature for underdialysis causes in America will now be better filled.

   In the second attempt to link statistics with acceptable medical logic, it should be stated clearly that patients can die from septicemia due to failure of sterilisation of a contaminated, reused dialyser. This risk is always present. Several incidents of such events having been reported in the literature [14, 15]. In both reports, a common water bacteria, *Mycobacterium chelonei*, was responsible for deaths. In the Louisiana outbreak, formalin was the sterilant and 14 patients died from complications of *M chelonei septicemia*. In Fresno, California, 2/5 patients infected with *M chelonei* died. Renalin was the sterilant in this report.

   In addition, there has always been an increased incidence of pyrogen fever reported with reuse compared to single use [16, 17, 18, 19].

These points are of great medico-legal importance as there are no quality control requirements for sterility or apyrogenicity of reused dialysers. Furthermore, the reused dialyser acts as a trap binding endotoxin which cannot be rinsed out by aqueous solutions but requires plasma or whole blood to remove it from the membrane [20, 21]. Finally, a report has just been published showing significantly higher levels of peripheral blood mononuclear cell IL–1ra (inteleukin–1 receptor antagonist) to be present in patients treated chronically with reused dialysers compared to patients on CAPD or patients with preterminal chronic renal failure [22, 23].

Taken together, this evidence suggests that the patient exposed to reuse receives a chronic stimulus to his inflammatory system by the regular infusion of pyrogen and perhaps by the disturbance of the production of bacterial permeability increasing protein (BPI) [24], a product of granulocyte degranulation, which normally protects the monocyte from stimulation by endotoxin. Chemical or heat alteration of protein layering of the reused membrane may play a critical role in disturbing the balance between BPI and lipopolysaccharide binding protein (LBP) [24] which specifically delivers endotoxin to the CD14 receptor of the monocyte and activates the cytokine cascade.

As chronic activation of the cytokine cascade can cause cachexia, it is reasonable to suggest that the reuse procedure may contribute to the bioburden of hemodialysis and explain, in part, the malnutrition and hypoalbuminemia so often observed in the dialysis patient who is about to die in America today [25].

Thus, one may presume that shortening of dialysis time and the employment of reuse may interact to produce inadequate dialysis and an increase in patient mortality which may take up to 5 years to manifest. This could then be the explanation for the relative increase in mortality seen with reuse in the US. Under these conditions, one is entitled to pose the question, should a responsible civilised government permit reuse of hemodialysers today?

References

1. Held PJ, Brunner FP, Odaka M, Garcia JR, Port FK, Gaylin DS. Five year survival for end stage renal disease patients in the United States, Europe and Japan, 1982 to 1987. Am J Kid Dis 1990; 15: 451–457.
2. Shaldon S, Koch KM. Survival and adequacy in long term hemodialysis. Nephron 1991; 59: 353–357.
3. Alter MJ, Favero MS, Moyer LS, Bland LA: National surveillance of dialysis-associated diseases in the United States, 1989. Trans Am Soc Artif Intern Organs 1991; 37: 97–109.
4. Fassbinder W, Brunner FP, Brynger H, Ehrich JHH, et al. Combined report on regular dialysis and transplantation in Europe, XX, 1989. Nephrol Dial Transplant 1991; 6 (Suppl 1): 5–35.
5. Held PJ, Wolfe RA, Gaylin DS, Port FK, Levin NW. Hemodialyzer reuse: disinfectant related mortality risk data. Oral presentation at American Society of Nephrology Baltimore November 16, 1992.
6. Held JP, Levin NW, Bovbjerg JD, Pauly MV, Diamond LH. Mortality and duration of hemodialysis treatment. J Am Med Ass 1991; 265: 871–875.

7. Farrell PC, Eschbach JW, Vizzo JE, Babb AL. Hemodialyser reuse: Estimation of area loss from clearance data. Kidney International 1974; 5: 446–450.
8. Ogden DA: Simultaneous reprocessing of hollow fiber dialyzers and blood tubing sets for multiple use. Dialysis and Transplantation 1974; 13: 366–375.
9. Garred LJ, Canaud B, Flavier JL, Poux C, Polito-Bouloux C, Mion C: Effect of reuse on dialyser efficacy. Artif Organs 1990; 14: 80–84.
10. Delmez JA, Weerts CA, Hasamear PD, Windus DW. Severe dialyser dysfunction undetectable by standard reprocessing validation tests. Kidney International 1989; 36: 478–484.
11. Saha LK, Van Stone JC, Differences between Kt/V measured during dialysis and Kt/V predicted from manufacturer clearance data. International J Artif Organs 1992; 15: 465–469.
12. Sargent JA. Shortfalls in the delivery of dialysis. Am J Kid Dis 1990; 15: 500–510.
13. Gotch FA, Yarian S, Keen M. A kinetic survey of US hemodialysis prescriptions. Am J Kid Dis 1990; 15: 511–515.
14. Bolan G, Reingold AI, Carson LA, Silcox VA, et al. Infections with mycobacterium chelonei in patients receiving dialysis and using processed dialysers. J Infect Dis 1985; 152: 1013–1019.
15. Lowry PW, Beck-Sague CM, Bland LA, Aguero SM, et al. Mycobacterium chelonei infection among patients receiving high-flux dialysis in a hemodialysis clinic in California. J Infect Dis 1990; 161: 85–90.
16. Gordon SM, Tipple M, Bland LA, Jarvis WR. Pyrogenic reactions associated with the reuse of disposable hollow fiber dialysers. J Am Med Ass 1988; 260: 2077–2081.
17. Beck-Sague CM, Jarvis WR, Bland LA, Arduino MJ, Aguero SM, Verosic G. Outbreak of gram-negative bacteremia and pyrogenic reactions in a hemodialysis center. Am J Nephrol 1990; 10: 397–403.
18. Alter MJ, Favero MS, Moyer LS, Bland LA. National surveillance of dialysis-associated diseases in the United States, 1989. Trans Am Soc Artif Intern Organs 1991; 37: 97–109.
19. Luft V, Schindler R, Lonnemann G, Shaldon S, Koch KM. Adsorption of exogenous pyrogen (EP) onto new and re-used high flux dialyzers (abstract). Nephrology Dialysis and Transplantation 1992; 7: 729.
20. Darbord JC, Decool A, Goury V, Vincent F. Biofilm model for evaluating hemodialyzer reuse processing. Dialysis & Transplantation 1992; 21: 644–649.
21. Dinarello CA. Interleukin–1 and tunor necrosis factor and their naturally occurring antagonists during hemodialysis. Kidney International 1992; 42 (Suppl 38): S68–S77
22. Pereira BJG, Poutsiaka DD, King AJ, Strom JA, Narayan G, Levey AS, Dinarello CA. In vitro production of Interleukin–1 receptor antagonist in chronic renal failure, continuous ambulatory peritoneal dialysis and hemodialysis patients. Kidney International 1992; 42: 1419–1424.
23. Marra MN, Thornton MB, Snable JL, Leong S, Lane J, Wilde CG, Scott RW. Regulation of the response to bacterial lipopoysaccharide by endogenous and exogenous lipopolysaccharide binding proteins. Blood Purification (in press).
24. Lowrie EG, Lew NL. Death risk in hemodialysis patients: The predictive value of commonly measured variables and an evaluation of death rate differences between facilities. Am J Kid Dis 1990; 15: 458–482.

CHAPTER 11

Survival and cardiovascular mortality in type I and type II diabetics with end stage renal disease

ANTHONY E.G. RAINE and EBERHARD RITZ

Introduction

Diabetic nephropathy is one of the most feared complications of diabetes, and is associated with a high prevalence of disability and total and cardiovascular mortality. In the past, access to renal replacement therapy (RRT) of patients with end stage renal failure due to diabetes has been restricted in Europe, particularly in those countries where there have been limitations on resources for provision of RRT [1]. However, changing treatment patterns over the years have resulted in an increase in acceptance of patients with diabetic nephropathy for RRT, from less than 2% of treated patients in Europe in 1974 [2] to over 10% in the mid–80's [3].

Despite the now widespread availability of RRT, survival of diabetic patients with end stage renal disease remains depressingly low. Studies in both the United States [4] and Europe [5] have shown that survival of diabetic patients is much lower than that of patients with end stage renal failure due to other causes. Moreover, the increase in mortality is largely due to an excess of cardiovascular death, in particular coronary heart disease [6].

Understanding of this problem is confounded by several issues; not least a lack of knowledge of the relative susceptibility of type I and type II patients with renal failure to cardiovascular complications. Type II diabetics are on average older than type I diabetics, and studies in non-uraemic patients have confirmed their high risk of vascular complications [7]. Although it was previously believed that in type II diabetics end stage renal failure rarely occurred [8], recent surveys have shown a high proportion of type II diabetics on RRT, both in the US [9] and in Europe [10]. Cohort studies have also shown that the rate of development both of proteinuria and of renal impairment from time of diagnosis is virtually identical in type I and type II diabetics [11].

Since 1965, the European Dialysis and Transplant Association (EDTA) has gathered annual information on patients receiving RRT in Europe. The purpose of the present report is to analyse the current survival in type I

E. A. Friedman (ed.), Death on Hemodialysis, 101–111.

and type II diabetics and non-diabetic patients commencing RRT in Europe between 1985 and 1990, in relation to age, sex and geographical distribution. Cardiovascular mortality rates in type I and type II diabetics have also been compared with those in non-diabetic RRT patients. In addition, these findings have been compared with those of a study of diabetic patients admitted to 28 German dialysis centres between January 1985 and October 1987, in whom patient outcome and predictors of cardiovascular death were examined [12].

Methods

The information recorded by the EDTA Registry on patients with end stage renal disease receiving RRT in Europe is updated annually on computer by returns made by all renal units in Europe for individual patients. Currently, over 2,400 centres in 36 countries report to the Registry. Information on cause of renal failure (primary renal disease) is coded for all patients, as is current mode of therapy. Patients with a primary renal disease given as diabetic nephropathy were selected for the present analysis. Up to 1982 a single code for diabetes was employed. Since 1983 separate codes have been employed for insulin dependent diabetes (type I) and for non-insulin dependent diabetes (type II). Responsibility for assigning the appropriate designation rests with the reporting physician. To compare current survival and mortality rates in type I and type II diabetic subgroups and in non-diabetics, analyses were performed on patients recorded as commencing all forms of renal replacement therapy between 1 January 1985 and 31 December 1990. The period of follow-up was up to five years, terminating at 31 December 1991.

For comparison with diabetic patients, patients with 'standard' primary renal diseases recorded by the EDTA Registry (chronic renal failure aetiology unknown, glomerulonephritis, pyelonephritis/interstitial nephritis, toxic nephropathies, cystic kidney diseases) [5] were analysed. For the present study this group is referred to as non-diabetic, but it should be emphasised that patients with hypertensive nephrosclerosis, vasculitides, other systemic diseases affecting the kidneys and other hereditary and metabolic renal diseases were excluded.

For calculation of mortality, two approaches have been used. First, actuarial survival analyses were performed on these patient groups as previously described [13]. Second, the cause-specific mortality rates per 1000 patient years at risk for patients with causes of death coded as ischaemic heart disease or cardiac arrest, cause unknown (sudden death) have been calculated by computing the exact time at risk of dying for each patient. The results presented are the average annual mortality rates for the first three years after commencing RRT. All data were stored and analysed using the Registry's VAX 750 computer (DEC) and software especially developed by Neville Selwood [14]. To enable comparison with this analysis based on the whole EDTA Registry population, data also included from a prospective study of 196 diabetic patients consecutively admitted to 28 German dialysis centres

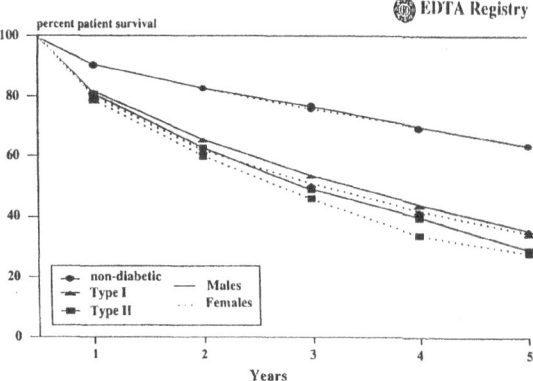

Fig. 1. Actuarial survival for all type I and type II diabetic and non-diabetic (standard primary renal diseases) males and females who began RRT in 1985–1990 (total Registry).

between January 1985 and October 1987. Classification of diabetes was made according to National Diabetes Data Group criteria [15]. By these criteria 67 patients were type I and 129 type II. Cardiovascular morbidity and mortality were assessed by annual follow-up. Blood pressure was measured as the average of 10 values obtained before the start of dialysis treatment, and echocardiographic analyses were performed according to a standardised protocol. Plasma samples obtained three months after commencing dialysis were analysed for cholesterol and lipoprotein subfraction [16].

Results

In the years 1985–1990, inclusive, a total of 13,888 type I diabetics (7,762 males, 6,126 females), 6,674 type II diabetics (3,665 males, 3,009 females) and 108,542 non-diabetic patients with standard primary renal diseases (63,442 males, 45,100 females) commencing RRT were enrolled with the EDTA Registry. Thus, approximately twice as many type I as type II diabetics were recorded as commencing treatment. However, it is likely that the proportion of type II diabetics has been under-estimated in these statistics, as patients with non-insulin dependent diabetes who were receiving insulin therapy may have been misclassified as having type I diabetes. This possibility is considered in more detail below.

Survival in diabetic and non-diabetic patients

Actuarial five year survival after commencing RRT for male and female type I and type II diabetic and non-diabetic patients is shown in Fig. 1. In non-diabetic patients, survival in males and females was almost identical, and was 77% at three years and 64% at five years for all ages together. Survival in diabetic patients was markedly poorer at all time points, and at five years was

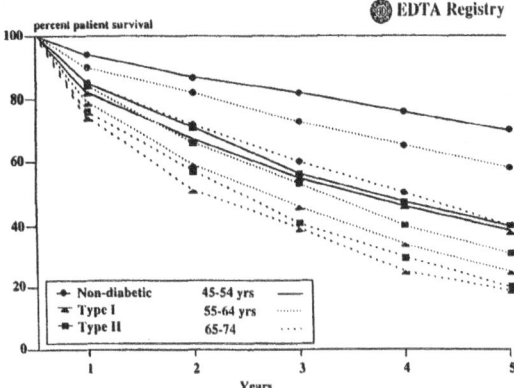

Fig. 2. Actuarial survival for all type I and type II diabetic patients and non-diabetic patients (standard PRD) who began RRT in 1985–1990, according to age at start of RRT.

approximately half that of non-diabetic patients. Survival was slightly lower in male and female type II diabetics, than type I diabetics.

The marginally lower overall survival in type II than type I diabetics is largely explained by their older age. A separate recent analysis has shown that the median age range of type II diabetic patients commencing RRT in Europe is the 65–74 year age group, in contrast to 55–64 years for type I diabetics [17]. To clarify the influence of age, actuarial survival in different age cohorts for both sexes in diabetic and non-diabetic patients was determined, and is shown in Fig. 2. It is apparent that for any age group, survival of type I diabetics is lower than that of type II diabetics. Because the type II diabetic population is older, all-ages survival curves for both forms of diabetes are similar (Fig. 1). It is clear also from Fig. 2. that survival of elderly non-diabetic patients aged 65–74 years remains higher than that of diabetic patients who are twenty years younger.

Recent reports from the EDTA Registry have shown that survival in patients on RRT is poorer in Northern than Southern Europe [18], and cardio-vascular mortality is higher [19]. It was therefore of interest to compare survival in diabetic and non-diabetic patients in 'Northern' European countries (Scandinavia and the United Kingdom) and 'Southern' European countries (Italy, France and Spain). Figure 3 illustrates the distinctly poorer five year survival in non-diabetic RRT patients in Northern Europe (63%) compared with that in Southern Europe (71%). However, five year survival in type I and type II diabetics from both Northern and Southern Europe was similar, and was markedly lower than that of non-diabetics, being approximately 40% in all groups.

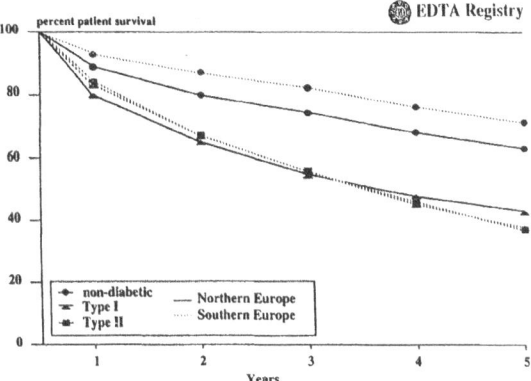

Fig. 3. Actuarial survival for type I and type II diabetic patients and for non-diabetic patients (standard PRD) commencing RRT in 1985–1990, in Northern Europe (Sweden, Norway, Finland, Denmark, United Kingdom) and Southern Europe (Italy, France, Spain). Date for type II diabetics from Northern Europe are not shown.

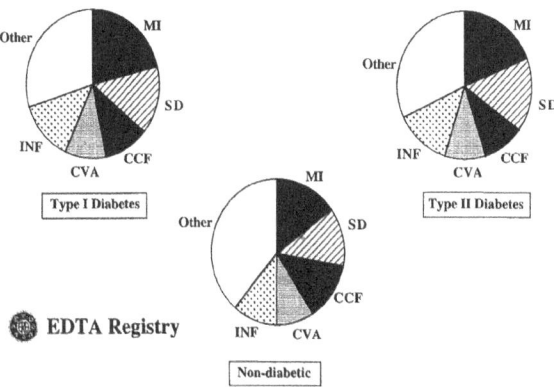

Fig. 4. Frequency of deaths due to specific cardiovascular causes and to infectious and other causes in male type I and type II diabetic patients and non-diabetic patients commencing RRT in 1985–1990 (total Registry). MI–myocardial infarction; SD–sudden death; CCF–congestive cardiac failure; CVA–cerebrovascular accident; INF–infection.

Cardiovascular mortality in diabetic and non-diabetic patients

The proportions of each patient group dying from different cardiovascular causes, from infectious causes and from other causes are shown for males in Fig. 4. Data for females were similar. Cardiovascular causes including stroke accounted for 57% of all deaths in type I diabetics and 55% of all deaths in type II diabetics, compared with 50% of deaths in non-diabetic patients. The proportion of deaths from stroke was similar in all three groups, whereas deaths from myocardial infarction and sudden death accounted for 36% of all deaths in type I diabetics and 35% in type II patients, compared with 28% in non-diabetics.

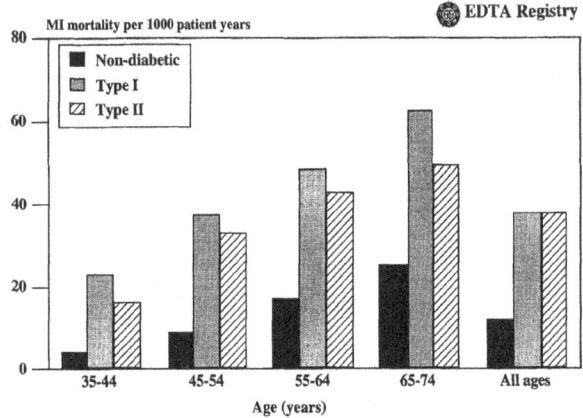

Fig. 5. Age-specific death rates from myocardial ischaemia and infarction in patients with type I and type II diabetic nephropathy and in non-diabetic patients (standard PRD) commencing RRT between 1985 and 1990

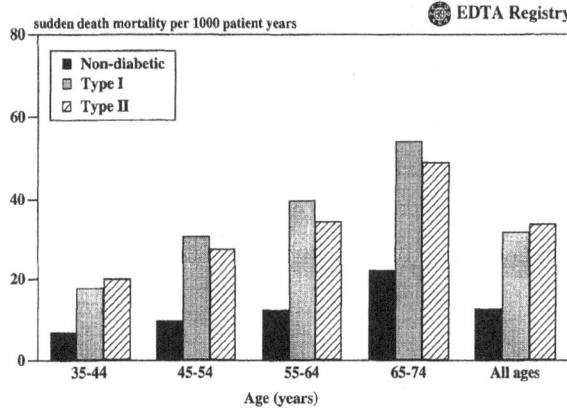

Fig. 6. Age-specific mortality rate from sudden death in type I and type II diabetic patients and in non-diabetic patients (standard PRD) commencing RRT between 1985 and 1990.

To quantify more accurately the differences in death rate from ischaemic heart disease, age-specific mortality rates from myocardial infarction and from sudden death (cardiac arrest) were compared in type I and type II patients and in non-diabetics (Figs. 5 and 6). As Fig. 5 shows, death rate from myocardial infarction was 4–5 times as great in young (35–44 year old) diabetics as in non-diabetics, and even in the older age cohorts (65–74 years), remained over twice as high in diabetics. Age-specific mortality from myocardial infarction was higher in type I diabetics in all age groups. However, because of the relatively greater number of elderly type II diabetics, all-ages mortality rate from myocardial infarction was identical in type I and type II diabetics at 38 per 1000 patient years (Fig. 5).

Sudden death, usually related to ischaemic heart disease or to electrolyte disorders, is also common in RRT patients, and particularly so in diabetics. As Fig. 6 shows, the age-specific mortality rates from sudden death in the diabetic and non-diabetic groups resembled those for myocardial infarction. Sudden death was three times as common in young diabetics as non-diabetics, and in each age group was more common in type I than type II diabetics, though when all ages were taken together, sudden death rate was similar in type I and type II patients. It is notable also that mortality rate from sudden death was only slightly lower than that documented as due to myocardial infarction; together, for all ages over seventy patients per 1000 diabetic RRT patients per year died from these two cardiac causes alone.

Risk factors for cardiac death in diabetic patients

Information on specific cardiovascular risk factors is not routinely recorded in the EDTA Registry database. The relationship between risk factors and cardiovascular outcome was addressed in the group of 196 dialysis patients entered in the German study group Diabetes and Uraemia, the results of which are presented in full elsewhere [12,16]. In this study, three year actuarial survival was again similar in type I (40%) and type II diabetics (43%) though slightly lower than in the overall EDTA diabetic cohort (Fig. 1). Cardiovascular causes of death again were very common, accounting for 62% of mortality in type I diabetics (52% from myocardial infarction and sudden death) and 60% in type II diabetics (31% from myocardial infarction and sudden death). Patients entering this study had uniformly severe hypertension; blood pressure greater than 160/95 mmHg was present in 98% of type I and 96% of type II diabetics, and median systolic blood pressure was 200 mmHg and diastolic blood pressure 100 mmHg. Severe left ventricular hypertrophy was also present (mean septal thickness 15 ± 4mm) [12]. No difference between patients dying of myocardial infarction or survivors was found with respect to blood pressure, left ventricular hypertrophy or diastolic dimension, though this lack of apparent relationship of these recognised risk factors to outcome may have been due to the rather uniform severity of both hypertension and target organ damage in the group studied [12]. No relationship was observed between cardiac death and indices of malnutrition, nor of insulin use [12].

In contrast, significant associations were observed with serum lipids. In type I diabetics, both total cholesterol (278 (224–293) vs 228 (148–329) mg/dl; $p < 0.005$) and LDL/HDL ratio (6.0 (5.3–8.6) vs 4.4 (2.4–8.3); $p <$ 0.05) were higher in patients dying of myocardial infarction than in survivors. Similarly in type II diabetics total and LDL cholesterol at start of RRT were also higher in patients dying of myocardial infarction or sudden death than in survivors (e.g. 177 (91–278) vs 154 (43–249) mg/dl for LDL cholesterol; p < 0.05).

Discussion

It is well known that the survival on RRT of patients with end stage renal disease due to diabetes is particularly poor [4,5], and that their cardiovascular mortality rate is especially high [5,6]. In non-uraemic diabetic patients the mortality from coronary artery disease is high in both type I [20] and type II patients [7]. The analyses reported here show that survival is equally impaired, and cardiovascular mortality equally increased, in both type I and type II diabetics with ESRD. However, some caution must be exercised in interpreting these analyses from the EDTA Registry database. It is very likely that relative under-reporting of the diagnosis of type II diabetes and over-reporting of type I diabetes has occurred as a consequence of attribution of patients with non-insulin dependent diabetes who are receiving insulin therapy to the category of type I disease. This likelihood is supported by the finding of the Diabetes in Uraemia study, in which 66% of the consecutive cohort of patients enrolled were type II [12], whereas EDTA Registry data show equal numbers of type I and type II diabetics on RRT in Germany [17]. Similarly, an Italian survey also describes 67% of patients undergoing RRT in Italy in 1987 as having type II diabetes [21]. In contrast, in Michigan, US, Cowie *et al.* showed that a majority of white patients on RRT had type I diabetes, but most black patients had type II disease [9].

Nevertheless, in both groups reported in the present study, the 1985–1990 EDTA cohort and the 1985–1987 German cohort, in which diabetes type was assigned by strict criteria, similar survival was observed in both type I and type II patients, implying that no major bias due to incorrect classification has arisen in the EDTA cohort. In both studies also, the similar survival in type I and type II patients despite the greater age of type II patients indicates that age-specific survival is lower in type I patients, as Fig. 2 confirms. Similarly, age-specific mortality for both myocardial infarction and sudden death is somewhat greater in type I patients than type II (Figs. 5 and 6), although all-ages mortality rate is equal for both types. For both diabetic types, age and cause-specific cardiovascular mortality is 3–6 fold higher than non-diabetic RRT patients, and is many times higher than that of the age and sex matched general population [22].

In non-diabetic RRT patients, major differences in survival and in cardiovascular mortality rate have been observed between Northern and Southern Europe, myocardial infarction death rate in particular being over four times higher in Northern Europe [19]. However, cardiovascular mortality in the general population is higher in Northern Europe, and in both Northern and Southern European countries a relatively constant 16–19 fold increase in mortality is present in RRT patients compared with the general population [19]. The implication is that in non-diabetic subjects the additional risk of ischaemic heart disease attributable to ESRD is superimposed on underlying fundamental differences in susceptibility to cardiovascular disease in the different general populations [19]. As the present analysis shows, these geographical differences disappear in type I and type II diabetic patients, survival in both Northern and Southern European patients being similar, and significantly poorer than in non-diabetics (Fig. 3). Thus, the major additional cardiovascular risk imposed by diabetes appears to obliterate the geographical differences in survival demonstrable in non-diabetics.

The precise reasons why diabetic patients, both uraemic and non-uraemic, develop such severe coronary artery disease remain uncertain. Manske *et al*, [23] have recently shown that in type I diabetic patients with ESRD significant coronary artery disease is present in the majority of patients older than 45, and is associated with hypertension, positive family history for ischaemic heart disease, reduced HDL cholesterol, and smoking. Atherosclerotic vascular disease in non-uraemic type II diabetic patients is related to atherogenic changes in lipoprotein composition typically present in this group, including reduced HDL cholesterol and increased total, LDL, and VLDL triglycerides [24]. The findings of the Diabetes and Uraemia study group [16] summarised here confirm the importance of dyslipidaemia as a risk factor for fatal myocardial infarction and sudden death in both type I and type II diabetics with end stage renal disease [16]. Taken together, these studies emphasise the need for controlled trials of lipid-lowering therapy to assess its utility in reducing the extreme levels of cardiovascular mortality present in diabetics with renal failure, whether insulin-dependent or non insulin-dependent.

Summary

Background

Although overall survival is poorer in diabetic than non-diabetic patients with end stage renal disease (ESRD), it is uncertain whether relative survival in type I or type II diabetics is worse, or whether mortality from ischaemic heart disease is greater in either sub-group. The factors predisposing to excessive cardiovascular mortality in these patients also remain uncertain. Actuarial survival and cause-specific cardiovascular mortality were therefore compared in type I and type II diabetics and non-diabetic patients on renal replacement therapy (RRT) in the EDTA Registry.

Methods

Cohorts of 13888 type I diabetics, 6674 type II diabetics and 108542 non-diabetic patients with standard primary renal diseases commencing RRT between 1 January 1985 and 31 December 1990 in Europe were analysed. Five year actuarial survival was determined, as was specific mortality rate from myocardial infarction and sudden death. For comparison, a group of 195 consecutive German diabetic patients is also reported, in whom RRT was commenced between 1985 and 1987, and in whom outcome in relation to cardiovascular risk factors was assessed.

Results

Overall five year survival was similar in type I and type II diabetics on RRT (36% vs 29%) and was only half that in non-diabetics (64%). Survival by age cohorts was lower in type I than type II patients. Five year survival was similar in type I and type II diabetics from Northern and Southern Europe, in contrast to the non-diabetic RRT population. Cardiovascular death accounted for 57% of deaths in type I diabetics and 55% in type II diabetics, compared with 50% in non-diabetic patients.

Age specific mortality rates for both myocardial infarction and for sudden death were 3–6 fold higher in diabetic than non-diabetic patients. In all age groups, the mortality rate was slightly higher in type I than type II diabetics. However, because of the preponderance of more elderly type II patients, all-ages mortality rate was equal for both myocardial infarction (38 per 1000 patient years) and sudden death (32 and 34 per 1000 patient years) in type I and type II patients.

Similar survival patterns and proportionate causes of cardiovascular death were present in a cohort of German type I and type II diabetic patients on RRT, in whom dyslipidaemia, in particular increased total cholesterol and raised LDL/HDL ratio, were significantly associated with fatal myocardial infarction.

Conclusions

As is the case for their risk of developing renal impairment, both type I and type II diabetics are at equal risk of developing fatal cardiovascular complications after commencing RRT. The exceptionally low survival and high mortality rate from ischaemic heart disease in these patients emphasises the need for controlled studies to assess the value of interventions, especially lipid lowering therapy.

Acknowledgement

We thank those doctors and their staff who have completed the question-naires which provided the data on which this report is based. Without their collaboration, this report would not have been possible.

References

1. Joint Working Party on Diabetic Renal Failure of the BDA, the Renal Association and the Research Unit of the Royal College of Physicians. Renal failure in diabetes in the UK: Deficient provision of care in 1985. Diabetic Med 1988; 5: 79–84.
2. Brunner FP, Giesecke B, Gurland HJ et al. Combined report on regular dialysis and transplantation in Europe, V, 1974. Proc Euro Dial Transp Assoc 1976; 12: 2–64.
3. Brunner FP, Brynger H, Challah S, et al. Renal replacement therapy in patients with diabetic nephropathy, 1980–85. Nephrol Dial Transplant 1988; 3: 585–595.

4. Vollmer WM, Wahl PW, Blagg CR. Survival with dialysis and transplantation in patients with end-stage renal disease. New Engl J Med 1903; 308: 1553–1558.
5. Brunner FP and Selwood NH. Results of renal replacement therapy in Europe, 1980–1987. Am J Kidney Dis 1990; 15: 384–396.
6. Brunner P and Selwood NH. Profile of patients on RRT in Europe and death rates due to major causes of death groups. Kidney Internationa 1992; 42 (Suppl 38): S4–S15.
7. Jarrett RJ. The epidemiology of coronary heart disease and related factors in the context of diabetes mellitus and impaired glucose tolerance. In Jarrett RJ Diabetes and Heart Disease, Amsterdam, Elsevier Science Publishers, editor., 1–23.
8. Ritz E, Nowack R, Flliser D, et al. Type II diabetes mellitus: is the renal risk adequately appreciated? Nephrol Dial Transplant 1991; 6: 679–682.
9. Cowie CC, Port FK, Wolfe RA, et al. Disparities in incidence of diabetic end-stage renal disease according to race and type of diabetes. N Engl J Med 1989 321: 1074–1079.
10. Catalano C, Postorino M, Kelly PJ, et al. Diabetes mellitus and renal replacement therapy in Italy: prevalence, main characteristics and implications. Nephro Dial Transplant 1990; 5: 788–796.
11. Hasslacher C, Ritz E, Wahl P and Michael C. Similar risks of nephropathy in patients with type I and type II diabetes mellitus. Nephrol Dial Transplant 1989; 4: 859–863.
12. Koch M, Thomas B, Tschöpe W, Ritz E. Survival and predictors of death in dialysed diabetics. Diabetologia (in press).
13. Brunner FP, Giesecke B, Gurland HJ, et al. Combined report on regular dialysis and transplantation in Europe, V, 1974. Proc Eur Dial Trans Assoc 1975; 12: 3–64.
14. Kramer P, Broyer M, Brunner FP, et al. Combined report on regular dialysis and transplantation in Europe, XIV, 1983. Proc Eur Dial Transplant Assoc Eur Ren Assoc 1905; 21: 2–68.
15. National Diabetes Data Group. Classification and diagnosis of diabetes mellitus and other categories of glucose intolerance. Diabetes 1979; 28: 1039.
16. Tschöpe W, Koch M, Thomas B, Ritz E. Serum lipids predict cardiac death in diabetic patients on maintenance hemodialysis (results of a prospective study). Nephron (in press).
17. Raine AEG. Epidemiology, development and treatment of end stage renal in non-insulin dependent diabetics in Europe. Diabetologia (in press).
18. Fassbinder W, Brunner FP, Brynger H, Raine AEG, et al. Combined report on regular dialysis and transplantation in Europe, XX. Nephrol Dial Transplant 1989; 6 (Suppl 1): 5–35.
19. Raine AEG, Margreiter R, Brunner FP, et al. Report on management of renal failure in Europe, XXII. Nephrol Dial Transplant 1992; 7 (Suppl 2): 7–35.
20. Krolewski AS, Kosinski EJ, Warram JH, et al. Magnitude and determinants of coronary artery disease in juvenile-onset, insulin-dependent diabetes mellitus. Am J Cardiol, 1987; 59: 750–755.
21. Catalano C, Postorino M, Kelly PJ et al. Diabetes mellitus and renal replacement therapy in Italy: prevalence, main characteristics and implications. Nephrol Dial Transplant 1990; 5: 788–796.
22. Brunner FP, Fassbinder W, Broyer M, et al. Combined report on regular dialysis and transplantation in Europe, XVIII, 1987. Springer Verlag, London, 1989; 5–31.
23. Manske MD, Wilson RF, Wang Y, Thomas W. Prevalence of, and risk factors for, angiographically determined coronary artery disease in type I diabetic patients with nephropathy. Arch Intern Med 1992; 152: 2450–2455.
24. Uusitupa, MD, Leo K, Niskanen MD, et al. 5-year incidence of atherosclerotic vascular disease in relation to general risk factors, insulin level, and abnormalities in lipoprotein composition in non-insulin dependent diabetic and nondiabetic subjects. Circulation 1990; 82: 27–36.

CHAPTER 12

Mortality comparison for diabetic ESRD patients treated with CAPD versus hemodialysis

FRIEDRICH K. PORT, CHRISTOPHER B. NELSON and
ROBERT A. WOLFE

Introduction

Selection of treatment options for patients with end stage renal disease (ESRD) has been a focus of much investigation. The treatment of patients with ESRD due to diabetic nephropathy falls primarily into three categories according to the United States Renal Data System Report [1] on prevalent patients treated as of December 31, 1990. Whereas, almost 1 in 5 patients had a functioning transplant, the dialysis group was treated primarily with center hemodialysis (82 percent) and CAPD (12 percent). Only 6 percent of diabetic dialysis patients were on other forms of peritoneal dialysis, home hemodialysis or unknown therapy. Diabetic patient survival following cadaveric renal transplantation was recently compared to that of transplant candidates on dialysis documenting superior outcomes for transplant recipients [2]. Comparative mortality risks according to selection of CAPD versus center hemodialysis (HD), however, have remained controversial and are the focus of this report specifically for patients with diabetic ESRD.

Methods

This study includes all adult patients with ESRD caused by diabetes who resided in Michigan and initiated dialysis therapy during the years 1980–89. Data were obtained from the files of the Michigan Kidney Registry (MKR) which contain demographic and longitudinal treatment information on all Michigan residents undergoing ESRD therapy independent of insurance status [3]. Due to the observed relatively high frequency of change in dialytic therapy during the first 4 months of ESRD [4], we arbitrarily assigned as 'treatment of choice' the therapy used on day 120 of ESRD. Patients under age 20 years, those with transplantation before day 120 and those of race other than white or black (2 percent) were excluded from this study. Study patients receiving

113

E. A. Friedman (ed.), Death on Hemodialysis, 113–119.
© 1994 *Kluwer Academic Publishers.*

Table 1. Demographic characteristics of the two
study groups

	Age 20–59	Age 60+
Total n	1458	985
Percent CAPD	36%	21%
Percent black	33%	42%
Percent female	46%	56%
Number of deaths	613	617

a transplant were censored (removed alive) on the day of transplantation.
In view of the probability of renal transplantation for the age group 20–60
years, this study population was separated into two age groups, ages 20–59
and above 60 years. Findings for the younger age group have been reported
previously [5] but are contrasted here with observations in older patients.

Statistical Methods: The Cox proportional hazards regression model was
used to estimate the relative mortality risk (RR) of CAPD patients relative
to HD patients [6]. This model adjusts for the influence of other independent
variables included in the model. In the following analyses, the mortality rates
of CAPD patients were compared with those of HD patients with adjustment
for age, race, sex and year of first ESRD (relative to 1989). An RR greater than
1 indicates a higher rate of death for CAPD as compared with the HD group,
an RR less than 1 indicates a lower rate, and an RR equal to 1 indicates no
difference in the death rates of the comparison and baseline groups. Ninety-
five percent confidence intervals reflect both the magnitude and precision of
the RR estimate. For the older age group the CAPD versus HD mortality risk
comparison was evaluated in specific age groups of interest using adjustments
for sex, race, year and their interactions in a stratified Cox model [6]. The
statistical analyses utilized the procedure PHREG of SAS v6.06 [7].

Results

This study includes 2443 patients with diabetic ESRD of whom 1458 were
of ages 20–59 and 985 over age 60 years at ESRD onset. Respectively 36
percent and 21 percent were classified as CAPD patients according to their
treatment on day 120 of ESRD. Other demographic characteristics are shown
in Table 1.

In both age groups the relative mortality risk (RR) was substantially and
significantly greater in white than in black patients when adjusting for covariates of age, sex, treatment modality and year of ESRD onset (Table 2). Males
also had a significantly higher mortality risk than females in the 20–59 year
age group when adjusting for other covariates including race. A later year of
ESRD start was significantly associated with lower mortality among CAPD
patients, but this finding was only statistically significant for the 20–59 year
age groups (for details see [5]). As expected, higher age at ESRD onset

Table 2. Relative mortality risk (Cox) by age, race, gender and year adjusted for treatment modality and to 1989

Covariate	Reference	Age 20–59	Age 60+
White	Black	1.44[b]	1.70[b]
Male	Female	1.22[a]	1.03
Age	per 10 years	1.14HD[b]; 1.37CAPD[b]	1.38[b]
Year of ESRD	per year	1.04HD; 0.91CAPD[b]	1.00

[a] $P < 0.05$; [b] $P < 0.01$

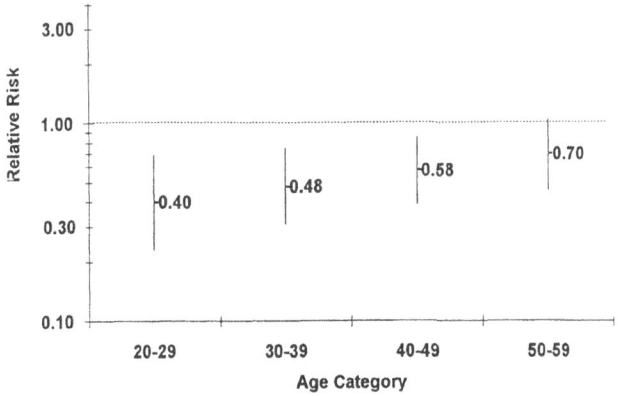

Fig. 1. Relative mortality risk (RR) for diabetic patients treated by CAPD compared to those treated by HD according to age groups below age 60 years. Vertical bars indicate the 5 to 95 % confidence intervals. Year of ESRD onset 1980–89 is adjusted to 1989. Other adjustments by the Cox model include race and gender. (Modifed from [5] with permission.)

was associated with higher mortality risk, however, the coefficient (or slope) for this correlation was significantly ($p = 0.03$) greater (steeper) for CAPD patients (RR = 1.37/10 yrs) than for HD patients (RR = 1.14/10 years) in the 20–59 age range. Among patients over age 60 years, the mortality risk increased by 38 percent per 10 years older at ESRD onset with similar slopes for CAPD and HD patients.

In view of the age by treatment interactions, results of the RR for CAPD compared to HD patients are reported by age group for 20–59 year old patients in Fig. 1. As previously reported, diabetic CAPD patients under age 50 years have substantially lower relative mortality risks than corresponding HD patients when adjusting for race, gender and year of ESRD onset to 1989. Results for ages 60 years and above are shown in Fig. 2. The age group of 65–74 years showed a 35 % higher mortality risk for patients treated by CAPD as compared to HD (RR = 1.35, p<0.02), whereas age groups 60–64 and 75<plus> years did not show a statistically significant difference in mortality

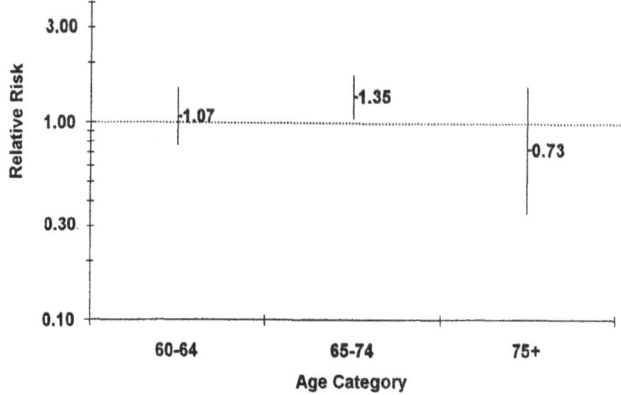

Fig. 2. Relative mortality risk (RR) for diabetic patients treated by CAPD compared to those treated by HD according to age groups above 60 years. Vertical bars indicate the 5 to 95 % confidence intervals. Adjustments by the Cox model include race, gender and year.

risk for the two treatment groups. The subgroups of ages 65–69 and 70–74 years had RR for CAPD compared to HD of 1.36 and 1.35 respectively. No statistical correlation for year of ESRD start and mortality risk was detected for ages over 60 years.

These RR estimates can be converted into survival probabilities by exponentiating the fraction of HD patients surviving with the RR to estimate the fraction of CAPD patients surviving. For example, if 40–49 year old hemodialysis patients have a one year survival of 80 percent, then the RR of 0.58 suggests a one year survival for CAPD patients of almost 88 percent $[0.80^{0.58} = 0.88]$. If the one year survival for 65–74 year old hemodialysis patients were 60 percent, then the RR of 1.35 would suggest a one year survival for CAPD patients of 50 percent.

Discussion

The present two studies from the Michigan Kidney Registry show that the statistically adjusted mortality risk (Cox) for diabetic CAPD patients is lower for ages 20–49 and higher for ages 65–74 than for corresponding HD patients. The magnitude of these risk differences is strikingly large with a 42–60 percent lower risk for 20–49 year old CAPD patients and a 35 percent higher risk for the 65–74 year age group on CAPD compared to HD. For younger patients (20–59 years) the risk difference described here for 1989 was in the opposite direction when previously described for 1980 [4]. This change occurred due to a crossing or reversal of relative risk near 1985–86 [5]. This gradual reversal is due to improving survival for CAPD patients (p = 0.001) and a trend towards worsening survival in HD patients (P<0.06). These trends over time (not observed for older patients) may be due to changes during the 1980s in dialytic therapy such as a decreasing dose of delivered hemodialysis and improving CAPD technologies. Alternatively, changes in selection to either modality could explain both trends if a selection of sicker patients away from CAPD and toward HD had gradually occurred during the 1980's.

Results from Italy [8] showed an age correlation for the CAPD versus HD mortality risk comparison that was in the opposite direction among all ESRD patients combined adjusting for diabetes. This observation may be related to differences in patient selection as demonstrated by the fact that CAPD patients in Italy are on average older than HD patients, whereas in the US they are on average younger.

An analysis from Spain [9] suggested poorer survival for CAPD than for HD patients; however when adjusting for diabetes status, age and cardiovascular disease the difference was not statistically significant. Again, older patients are more likely treated with CAPD in Spain, suggesting different selection characteristics compared to Michigan and the United States. A comparative study in the US by Serkes *et al.* [10] found for diabetic ESRD patients no statistically significant difference in patient survival. The present study has the advantage over these studies of having a larger sample size, being population based rather than research center based and focusing specifically on diabetic ESRD.

The US Renal Data System (USRDS) also studied the relative mortality risk for patients with diabetes by dialytic modality (from day 90 of ESRD) using the Cox analysis. When adjusting for demographic and comorbidity covariates, the mortality risk was overall significantly higher for CAPD patients (RR = 1.28) than for HD patients [11]. This comparison described the finding at the average age of 58 years. There appeared to be trends for a larger adverse outcome for CAPD patients above this age and a smaller risk difference below this average age compared to the corresponding HD group. The advantage of this USRDS study was the statistical adjustment for comorbid conditions.

For ages <60 years this USRDS case mix study documented slightly but significantly fewer comorbid conditions among diabetic CAPD than HD patients [12]. If this finding applied also to Michigan patients, then the difference between young CAPD and HD patient mortality risk would be somewhat reduced by such an adjustment. If, on the other hand, the time trends observed in Michigan of improving outcomes in CAPD patients of this age group applied to the United States, then the USRDS results for 1986–87 incident patients would extrapolate to a larger benefit for CAPD outcomes by 1989, the reference year of the Michigan study. Thus, the results of the USRDS and Michigan studies appear to agree qualitatively.

A possible reason for the differences in results for younger versus older patients may relate to the fact that younger diabetic ESRD patients have primarily type I insulin dependent diabetes [13] which may have different disease specific outcomes than those for type II diabetics.

Mortality risk assessment by treatment modality can address the comparison of the treatment itself by censoring when the patient changes to another treatment modality (or after a 30 day carry-over period) as a treatment history analysis. Alternatively, it can focus on the intent-to-treat to provide information to the clinician and patient for the decision of the early treatment of choice. This latter approach which censored patients only on the day of renal transplantation but not at change in dialytic modality, was used in the Michigan studies described above. When employing the treatment history analysis, censoring at transplantation and 30 days after change in dialytic modality, the risk differences for CAPD versus HD patients were very similar to those described above [5]. Among nondiabetic patient groups, both types of analyses from Michigan [5] and the USRDS [11] gave mortality risk results that were not statistically different for CAPD and HD patients.

Conclusion

Diabetic CAPD patients aged 65–74 years had higher mortality risk than corresponding HD patients. By contrast, in the late 1980s young diabetic CAPD patients (age 20–49) had lower mortality risk than similar HD patients. These results may be due to the dialytic treatment itself or to unmeasured severity indicators of comorbidity or other unrecognized selection criteria. Future research needs to address such potential factors in prospective studies.

Acknowledgment

This work was supported in part through a grant from the Baxter Extramural Grants Program.

References

1. United States Renal Data System: USRDS 1993 Annual Data Report. National Institutes of Health, National Institute of Diabetes and Digestive and Kidney Diseases, Bethesda MD, March 1993.
2. Port FK, Wolfe RA, Mauger EA, Berling DP, Jiang K. Comparison of survival probabilities for dialysis patients versus cadaveric renal transplant recipients. JAMA 1993 (in press).
3. Port FK, Cord EC. Michigan Kidney Registry Report of Progress. Ann Arbor MI: MKR, 1992: 1–69.
4. Wolfe RA, Port FK, Hawthorne VM, Guire KE. A comparison of survival among dialytic therapies of choice: in-center hemodialysis vs continuous ambulatory peritoneal dialysis at home. Am J Kidney Dis 1990; 15: 433–440.
5. Nelson CB, Port FK, Wolfe RA, Guire KE. Comparison of CAPD and hemodialysis patient survival with evaluation of trends during the 1980s. J Am Soc Nephrol 1992; 3: 1147–1155.
6. Cox DR. Regression models and life tables (with discussion). J R Stat Soc 1972; 34: 197–220.
7. SAS Institute INC. SAS/STAT Software. The PHREG procedure preliminary documentation. Release 6.06. Cary, NC; SAS Institute Inc; 1991.

8. Maiorca R, Vonesh EF, Cavalli P, et al. A multicenter, selection-adjusted comparison of patients and technique survivals on CAPD and hemodialysis. Perit Dial Int 1991; 11: 118–127.

9. Gentil MA, Carriazo A, Pavón MI, Rosado M, Castillo D, Ramos B, Algarra GR, Tejuca F, Bañasco VP, Milan JA. Comparison of survival in continuous ambulatory peritoneal dialysis and hospital haemodialysis: A multicentric study. Nephrol Dial Transplant 1991; 6: 444–451.

10. Serkes KD, Blagg CR, Nolph KD, Vonesh EF, Shapiro F. Comparison of patient and technique survival in continuous ambulatory peritoneal dialysis (CAPD) and hemodialysis: A multicenter study. Perit Dial Int 1990; 10: 15–19.

11. Held PJ, Port FK, Turenne MN, Gaylin DS, Hamburger RJ, Wolfe RA. Continuous ambulatory peritoneal dialysis and hemodialysis: A comparison of patient mortality with adjustment for comorbid conditions. JAMA 1993 (in press).

12. US Renal Data System. Patient selection to peritoneal dialysis versus hemodialysis according to comorbid conditions. Am J Kidney Dis 1992; 20(Suppl 2): 20–26.

13. Cowie CC, Port FK, Wolfe RA, Savage PJ, Moll PP, Hawthorne VM. Disparities in incidence of diabetic end-stage renal disease according to race and type of diabetes. N Engl J Med 1989; 321: 1074–1079.

CHAPTER 13

The relative contribution of measured variables to death risk among hemodialysis patients[*]

E.G. LOWRIE, W.H. HUANG, N.L. LEW and Y. LIU

Introduction

Each year, as part of its Quality Improvement and information sharing activities, National Medical Care (NMC) evaluates possible factors contributing to death risk among patients treated in its affiliated centers focusing on data gathered during the preceding year. We hope in this way to detect clinically relevant risk trends as they respond to changing clinical practice. The purpose of this article is to summarize data collected during 1991 and compare them with past analyses of similar sort.

The analysis enhances our past efforts because the model building strategy was changed slightly. The purpose was to better understand the nature of the statistical models and to gain insight into the way variables interact during the model building process. We also added routine and other laboratory variables which we had not hitherto included in the models. Hepatic enzymes, serum sodium, hematocrit, and the like were among those variables. We also evaluated non-laboratory data such as blood pressure, weight, and so forth in a subset of our patients.

The data provide more support for the critical nature of good nutrition and adequate dialysis intensity for the well-being of patients. There are new findings, however. The anion gap appears to be a significant risk factor in our patients but the interpretation of its value is complicated. Briefly, a normal anion gap, like a low BUN, means nothing if the patient is undernourished. But, in the presence of adequate nutrition high anion gap is a significant risk factor. There are a number of other findings – some new, some old – and we will touch on a few. For example, the body burden of aluminum appears to be a continuing risk for patients in spite of all the attention it has received during recent years. And increased risk starts at very low concentrations. Finally, we

---

[*] This article has been abstracted from a technical memorandum to NMC Medical Directors dated February 26, 1993.

E. A. Friedman (ed.), Death on Hemodialysis, 121–141.
© 1994 *Kluwer Academic Publishers.*

believe that the data about both blood pressure and hematocrit will stimulate both comment and controversy.

Analysis Strategy

Patients receiving 3 weekly hemodialyses treatments on January 1, 1991 who were either still receiving dialysis on December 31, 1991 or had died were included in the analysis. Earlier analytic strategies used a two phase process [1, 2]. First, logistic regression [3] techniques were used to identify 'case mix' predictors of death such as age, sex, race, diabetic status, and renal diagnosis. Predictors found significant were fixed in the statistical model. Selected laboratory variables were then added to it in a second phase. Risk profiles for laboratory predictors which were found to be significant were then constructed. The effect of adding laboratory variables on the risk profile for the case mix predictors was also evaluated [4].

We changed the strategy this time by omitting the first phase selection of case mix related predictors. Instead, all variables – both laboratory and case mix – were made available to a forward stepwise logistic regression program in a 'one phase' strategy.

Forward stepwise selection programs proceed by first selecting that variable which is most closely associated with death risk – the one with the highest Chi-square χ^2 statistic. That variable is selected by the program for inclusion in the model. Next, the odds of death are adjusted for that (selected) variable and new χ^2 values are computed for the remaining variables. Those variables are then examined to determine the one associated with the highest χ^2 and it is selected for inclusion in the model. For example, suppose that both serum creatinine concentration and the URR* have high-χ^2 values and are correlated with each other. Suppose also that serum creatinine concentration is selected in the first step. χ^2 values are computed for URR and all other variables at a constant value of serum creatinine. The variable with the highest χ^2 – URR in our example – is then selected for inclusion at this second step. Next, all remaining variables are adjusted for the first 2 and the one most closely associated with death risk is selected for inclusion in Step 3. The process continues until no other variables are associated with death probability at some specified level of statistical significance – $p \leq .05$, for example.

We added a number of routinely measured but not previously considered laboratory variables to the base analysis this year. Serum sodium, chloride, ferritin, LDH, bilirubin, SGOT, and so forth were numbered among them. In addition, variables such as PTH, serum aluminum concentration, ionized calcium, and so forth are not determined routinely on all patients but are available on a significant subset. They also were analyzed in a second stage strategy by adding them one at a time to the Base Model. Finally, a separate

---

* URR means Urea Reduction Ratio and is computed as $100 \times (1 - ((\text{Pre-dialysis BUN} - \text{Post-dialysis BUN})/\text{Pre-dialysis BUN}))$.

Table 1. Mortality analysis, 1991 data case mix & laboratory predictors[a]
(includes anion gap)

Variables	Entry χ^2	Final model[b]		
		Odds ratio	χ^2	p
Creatinine (mg/dl)	662.6	0.841	283.98	0.0001
URR (%)	301.3	0.952	198.09	0.0001
Albumin (gm/dl)	205.1	0.396	114.59	0.0001
Anion gap	239.8	1.072	36.34	0.0001
Age (yrs)	145.1	1.029	210.46	0.0001
Bilirubin (mg/dl)	84.7	2.021	31.57	0.0001
LDH (u/l)	51.6	1.003	42.90	0.0001
Sex (ref = male)	45.6	0.745	33.62	0.0001
Sodium (meq/l)	40.5	0.975	4.47	0.0344
WBC (1000/mcl)	18.8	1.045	15.38	0.0001
Ferritin (ng/ml)	15.6	1.000	16.58	0.0001
Phosphorus (mg/dl)	14.4	1.065	20.38	0.0001
Calcium (mg/dl)	16.0	1.125	13.47	0.0002
Cholesterol (mg/dl)	12.0	0.998	11.41	0.0007
HCT (%)	10.0	0.985	5.49	0.0191
Protein (g/dl)	9.6	0.849	13.99	0.0002
Glomerulonephritis	9.0	0.720	14.04	0.0002
Obs. uropathy	7.0	0.517	7.79	0.0053
Diabetes (ref = non-diabetic)	7.4	0.865	8.34	0.0039
Iron (mcg/dl)	6.6	0.997	7.14	0.0076
SGOT (u/l)	5.4	1.004	3.84	0.0500
Cystic kidney disease	5.1	0.722	5.15	0.0232
Chloride (meq/dl)	4.5	0.974	5.87	0.0154
Uric acid (mg/dl)	4.6	1.048	4.76	0.0291
Alk phos (u/l)	4.2	1.000	4.23	0.0400

[a] $N = 16,153$; Total model $\chi^2 = 2019.45$; $R^2 = 0.1367$.
[b] Non-significant variables: race, collagen vascular disease, multiple myeloma, renal failure of unspecified cause, BUN, CO_2, K, HBsAg, SGPT, Triglyceride

database contains determinations of blood pressure, body weight, and so forth. We used a second logistic regression process, patterned after the Base Analyses, to evaluate case mix, laboratory, and these new potential death risk predictors in that subset of patients.

Results

The base model

Table 1 shows the death risk predictors in order of their selection by the forward stepping logistic process. The χ^2 at entry into the model, odds of death, χ^2 in the final model, and its associated p value are shown.

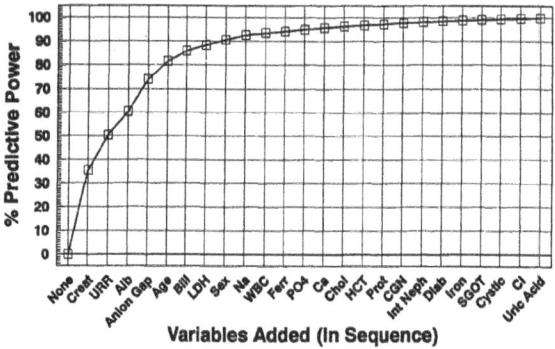

Fig. 1. Percent of final logistic model predictive power as variables are added sequentially to it.

Serum creatinine was selected first. The χ^2 at initial selection was 663. The initial χ^2 associated with albumin was 626. Hence, the association of creatinine and albumin with death risk, prior to any statistical adjustment, were nearly equal. Serum creatinine and serum albumin were directly (and highly) correlated ($r = 0.37$; $p < .001$). Hence, the χ^2 associated with albumin was reduced ($\chi^2_{albumin} = 258$) during the second stage of the model building process. Because URR and creatinine are inversely correlated ($r = -0.27$; $p < .001$), χ^2_{URR} increased from 107 to 301 during this second stage. Therefore, URR was selected at Step 2 and serum albumin concentration was then selected at Step 3.

Although serum albumin concentration was selected first in some models used with these and other data sets, serum creatinine, URR, and serum albumin are always the first 3 variables selected as being most closely associated with death risk. The odds ratio for each variable is always less than one so low values for each are associated with greater risk.

Anion gap* is always associated with higher odds of death after statistical adjustment for albumin, URR, and creatinine. Serum sodium concentration is a significant but weak predictor even after adjusting for anion gap but it is low sodium which is associated with greater risk. Low chloride, like low sodium, is associated with greater death risk as suggested by $Odds_{cl} = 0.974$.

Variables possibly reflecting liver disease such as LDH, SGOT and bilirubin are finding their way into these models. The presence of the HbsAg marker was not associated with death risk.

Figure 1 shows how the predictive power of this statistical model develops as variables are added to it. The Y-Axis shows the cumulative fraction of the final models predictive power estimated by ratio of the model χ^2 at that point in the stepping process to the final model χ^2.

The combination of creatinine, URR, and albumin contribute about 60% of this model's power. Adding anion gap contributes another 13%. The combined variables of creatinine, URR, albumin, anion gap, and age, contribute slightly

---

* We computed Anion Gap thusly: $AG = (Na + K) - (Cl + CO_2)$.

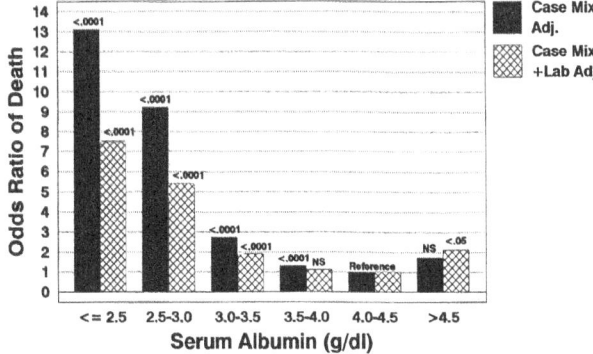

Fig. 2.   Risk profile for serum albumin.

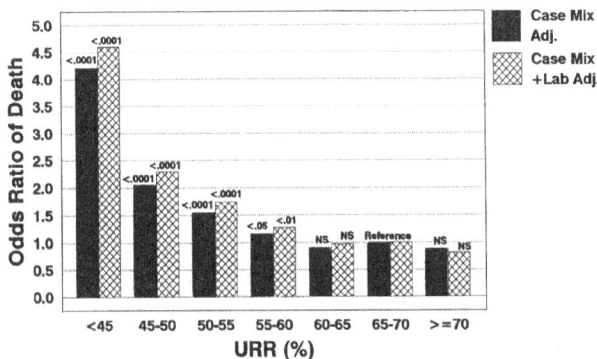

Fig. 3.   Risk profile for urea reduction ratio (URR).

over 80% of this model's predictive power. Adding bilirubin, LDH, and gender leads us to observe that 8 variables contribute 90% of this model's final predictive power. The remaining 16 variables contribute the final 10%. Hence, 1/3 of the variables contribute 90% of the power. Such observations may serve to focus the attention of physicians and investigators on particular problems as they set priorities for their various clinical and research activities.

The big 3: albumin, URR, and creatinine

These 3 variables, taken together, are the most important associates of death risk. Figure 2 shows the risk profile for serum albumin concentration. The odds of death at different albumin concentrations is compared to the reference concentration which was 4.0–4.5 gm/dl. Odds ratios adjusted for case mix variables (age, sex, race, diabetic status, and baseline renal disease) and also adjusted for those variables plus the other significant laboratory predictors are shown. Earlier analyses [1, 2, 5] have also suggested that death risk increases rapidly with decreasing serum albumin concentration.

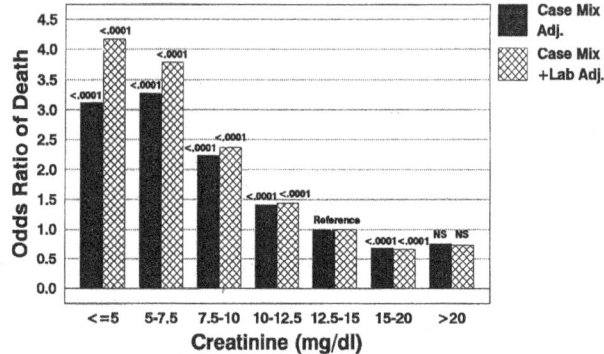

Fig. 4.   Risk profile for serum creatinine concentration.

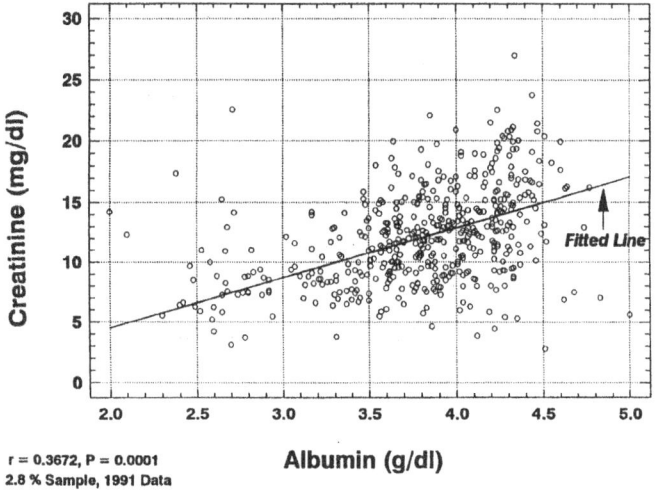

Fig. 5.   The relationship between serum creatinine and serum albumin concentration ($r = 0.37$; $p < .001$).

Figure 3 is a plot of similar format showing relative death risk as a function of URR. Values below 60% are clearly associated with increased risk. We have described similar findings in the past [5].

Figure 4 shows the risk profile for serum creatinine concentration. The odds of death increase at lower concentrations and this is true up to serum creatinine concentrations of about 20 mg/dl.

The relationships among albumin, URR, and creatinine are complex [2]. Figure 5 shows the relationship between serum albumin and serum creatinine concentrations. It is direct and highly significant and has been reported before [4]. Albumin concentration is thought to reflect visceral protein mass. Creatinine concentration will depend in part upon the generation rate of creatinine from the body's muscle mass. Higher generation rates, and therefore

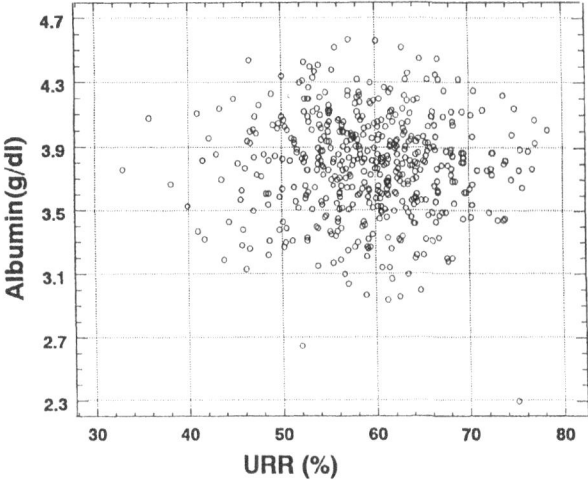

Fig. 6.   The relationship between serum albumin concentration and URR. There is no significant correlation.

higher concentrations, will reflect greater muscle mass all else being equal. The correlation between serum albumin concentration and serum creatinine concentration in these persons with compromised creatinine elimination is therefore easy to understand because the adequacy of visceral and somatic protein stores is likely correlated.

Figure 6 shows the relationship between URR and serum albumin concentration. Simply stated, there is none ($r = -.013; p = $NS).

Figure 7 shows the relationship between URR and serum creatinine concentration. It is inverse so that high URR is associated with low creatinine. Creatinine clearance is one measure of dialyzer efficiency so this relationship is easy to understand. However, high creatinine is associated with better survival than low and so is high URR. Does the correlation suggested by Fig. 7 mean that higher URR actually places patients at greater risk because it lowers creatinine? That is not likely but this relationship does illustrate the complex nature of interpreting the meaning of creatinine concentration in dialysis patients.

Our attempt to simplify clinical interpretation of the relationships among creatinine, albumin, and URR is illustrated by Fig. 8. Three planes reflecting creatinine concentrations of 6 mg/dl, 12, and 18 are shown at various values of URR and serum albumin concentration. At all values of creatinine, death probability falls rapidly as URR increases and this is particularly true at the lower levels of serum albumin concentration. Similarly, death probability falls as albumin increases at all values of URR. Finally, the death probability differences between creatinine concentrations are minimum when both albumin and URR are high.

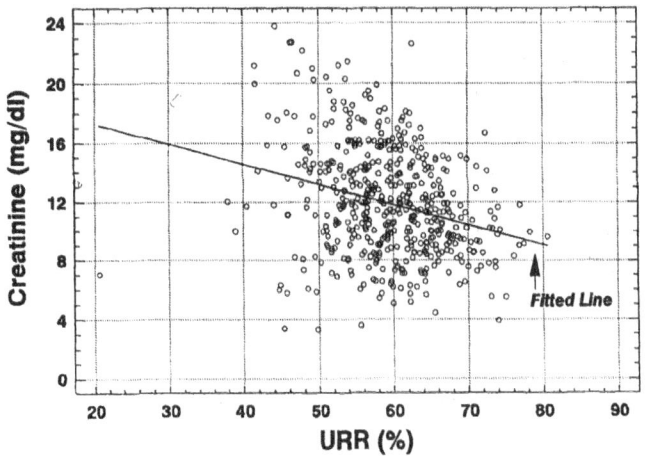

Fig. 7.   The relationship between serum creatinine concentration and URR ($r = 0.275$; $p < .001$).

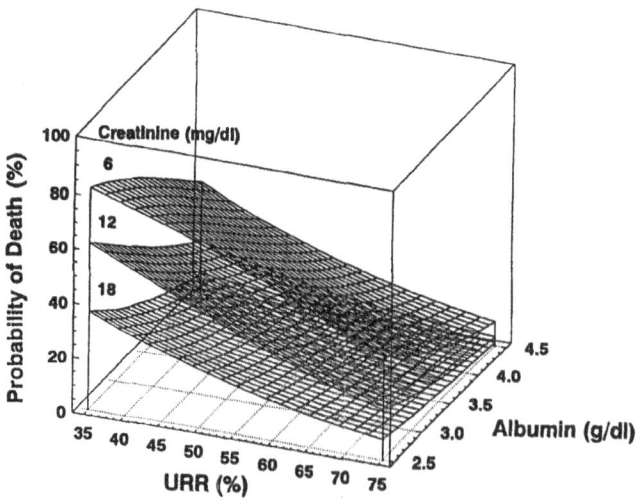

Fig. 8.   Death probability during one year is shown as a function of the joint values of URR, serum albumin concentration, and serum creatinine concentration.

To the clinician this figure says that death risk is minimized when URR, albumin, and creatinine are high. If albumin and URR are high the death risk difference between creatinine concentrations is minimized. Therefore, the clinician can probably ignore the complicated character of serum creatinine concentration, which reflects elements of both nutrition and dialysis intensity, and use it simply for supplementary information if albumin and URR are known.

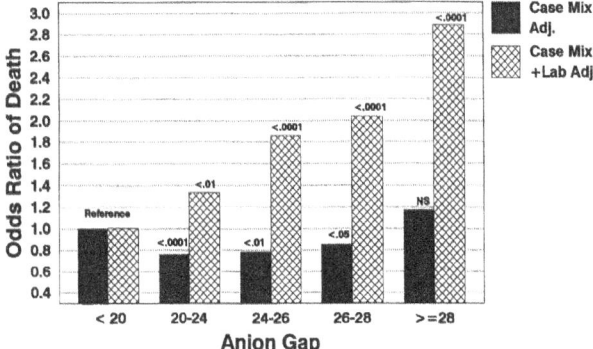

Fig. 9.   Risk profile for anion gap.

Table 2. Biochemical correlates* of the anion gap (N = 17,500 ±)

Variables	r	p
Phosphorus (mg/dl)	0.482	<.001
Creatinine (mg/dl)	0.435	<.001
BUN (mg/dl)	0.429	<.001
Albumin (gm/dl)	0.276	<.001
Uric acid (mg/dl)	0.210	<.001
PTH (intact) (pg/ml)	0.193	<.001
Aluminum (mcg/dl)	0.159	<.001
CO_2^c (meq/l)	−0.487	<.001
Chloride^c (meq/l)	−0.302	<.001
Potassium^c (meq/l)	0.326	<.001

* $r \geq 0.15$ included
^{c} = Calculation variable
r $(Na^c) = 0.06$

Anion Gap

Figure 9 shows the risk profile for anion gap. Prior to adjusting for the laboratory values, increasing anion gap was associated with reduced odds of death until anion gap exceeded about 26 meq/L. Compared to the reference range (anion gap < 20), $Odds_{AG=20--24} \approx 0.78$ prior to adjustment for other laboratory variables. That means the higher anion gap was associated with a *risk benefit*. After adjustment for laboratory variables $Odds_{AG=20--24} \approx 1.35$ and increasing anion gap was associated with progressively increasing odds of death.

    We evaluated this interesting observation in two ways. First we determined the biochemical correlates of anion gap. Table 2 shows the results. Serum phosphorous was directly correlated with anion gap so that high phosphorous was associated with high anion gap. BUN, creatinine, and albumin were also directly correlated with anion gap. All 3 may reflect the nutritional

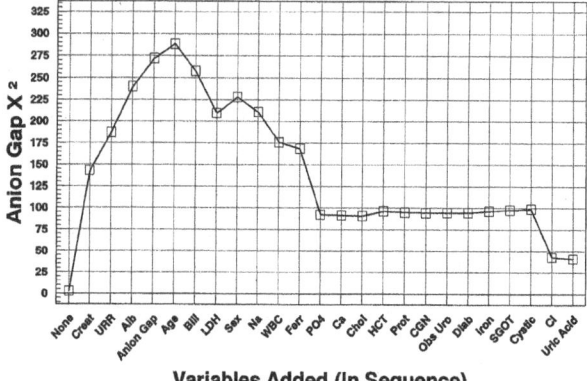

Variables Added (In Sequence)

Fig. 10.   The evolution of X^2 anion gap as a function of adjustment for other variables in a logistic model.

status of patients' high values of each substance being associated with better nutrition. While albumin, like PO_4 is an anion, its association with anion gap may be due more to joint effect of inadequate nutrition on both albumin concentration and 'unexplained' anion production (reduces it) than on the fact that albumin carries a negative charge. The reason for this interpretation is implied by Fig. 10 which will be discussed in the next paragraph. Anion gap was also associated statistically with uric acid, intact PTH, and serum aluminum concentration. We will not comment on the association of CO_2, chloride, and potassium because the values are included in calculating the gap.

We also traced the evolution of the χ^2 anion gap as variables were included in the statistical model. Figure 10 shows the result. Prior to adjusting for serum creatinine concentration, χ^2 anion gap is quite low (χ^2 anion gap = 2.9; $p = .09$). After adjustment for creatinine (so that association of anion gap with the odds of death is evaluated at the same creatinine level) χ^2 anion gap increases remarkably. Adjustment for URR and albumin increase it even more so that it is the highest of all remaining variables at Step 4 and is therefore selected for inclusion in the model. Adjustment for other variables reduces χ^2 anion gap somewhat decrease is sharp when PO_4 is added to the model. Unlike adjustment for albumin which increases χ^2 anion gap adjustment for PO_4 reduces it. We observe a similar phenomenon when Cl is added to the model. The downward adjustment for PO_4 and Cl probably occur because both are anions, one of which is included in the computation of anion gap. The adjustment is upward when albumin is added to the model, however. This observation leads us to believe that the correlation between albumin and anion gap results more from the joint effect of nutrition on albumin and anion production than it does from albumin's negative charge.

These analyses suggest that better nutritional status is associated with greater anion gap. We speculate that hydrogen ion and unexplained anion generation are in part functions of protein intake. Poor nutrition would therefore

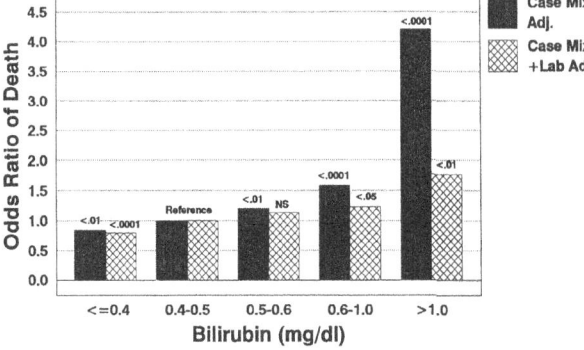

Fig. 11.   Risk profile for serum bilirubin concentration.

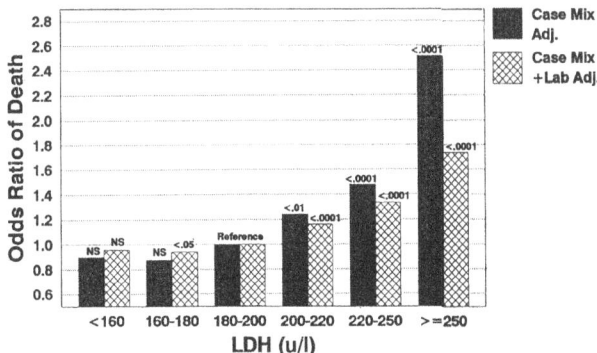

Fig. 12.   Risk profile for LDH.

be associated with low anion generation and anion gap. Prior to considering the nutrition of the patient, therefore, anion gap is not, in and of itself, strongly correlated with death risk. If anything, elevated anion gap is associated with a moderate risk benefit – probably because it is associated with better nutrition. Once nutritional status is held constant, however, the deleterious effect of these unexplained anions is revealed by the risk profile. The preliminary message, we believe, is that one should feed patients to assure good nutrition, dialyze them aggressively (URR) to remove the waste, and assure adequate repletion of their body buffers.

LDH, bilirubin, and the hepatic variables

Figures 11 and 12 show the risk profiles for bilirubin and LDH respectively. In the case mix plus lab adjusted models LDH has been adjusted for bilirubin and SGOT (as well as other laboratory variables) while bilirubin has been adjusted for LDH, SGOT, and other variables. In general, LDH values over the 180–200 u/l are associated with greater odds of death. Risk seems to increase progressively with serum bilirubin concentration, at least for values > 0.4 mg/dl. These predictors are certainly not as powerful as creatinine,

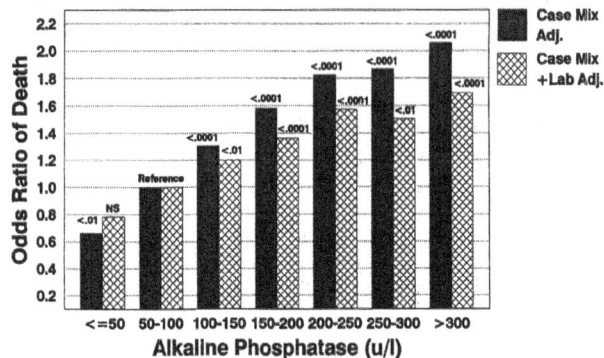

Fig. 13.   Risk profile for alkaline phosphatase.

URR, albumin, anion gap or age but are nonetheless associated highly with death probability among our patients. Furthermore, the levels of bilirubin and LDH which are associated with increased death risk are not that strikingly high.

LDH was associated directly with serum bilirubin ($r = .17; p < .001$) and SGOT ($r = 0.36; p < .001$) as well as SGPT ($r = .22; p < .001$). LDH was also directly correlated with anion gap ($r = 0.14; p < .001$) but inversely correlated with total calcium ($r = -0.24; p < .001$) and ionized calcium ($r = -.16; p < .001$). LDH does correlate directly but weakly with serum phosphorous ($r = .12; p < .001$). Serum bilirubin which correlates with LDH, SGOT ($r = 0.27; p < .001$) and SGPT ($r = 0.10; p < .001$) correlates also with ferritin ($r = .014; p < .001$) and serum iron ($r = 0.15; p < .001$).

Other routine laboratory variables

Figure 13 shows the risk profile for alkaline phosphatase which is a weak predictor (χ^2 alk phos $= 4.4$) in the overall model. High alkaline phosphatase is associated with greater death risk.

Figure 14 shows the risk profile for serum phosphorous. Both low and high levels of phosphorous are associated with increased death risk both before and after adjustment for laboratory variables. This finding is similar to earlier observations [1].

We include the risk profile for serum sodium as Fig. 15. Note that before adjustment for other laboratory variables low sodium is a significant predictor.

Hematologic variables

Figure 16 shows the risk profiles for white blood count. We have not evaluated this observation in detail but note that white count before adjustment for laboratory values is a significant predictor but it becomes weak after adjustment.

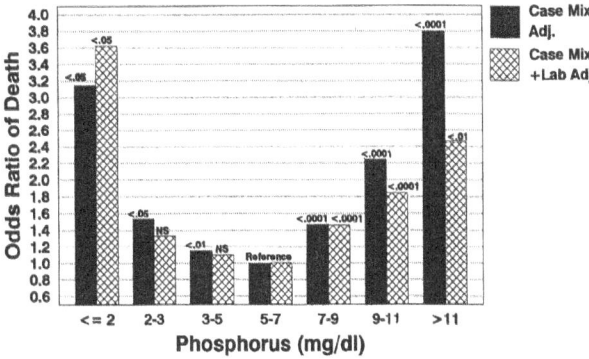

Fig. 14.   Risk profile for serum phosphorous concentration.

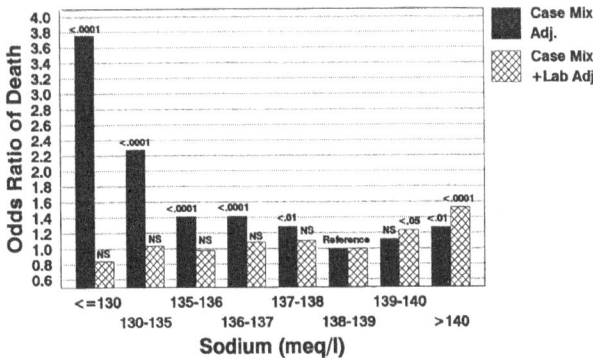

Fig. 15.   Risk profile for serum sodium concentration.

Figure 17 shows the risk profile for hematocrit. The risk profile is U-shaped. Compared to the reference range of 30–35 vol%, both high and low hematocrit are associated with greater risk. Adjustment for laboratory variables produces only minor effect except when hematocrit is very low.

We have not evaluated the reasons for the adjustment in those patients with low hematocrit nor can we explain why risk appears to *increase* when

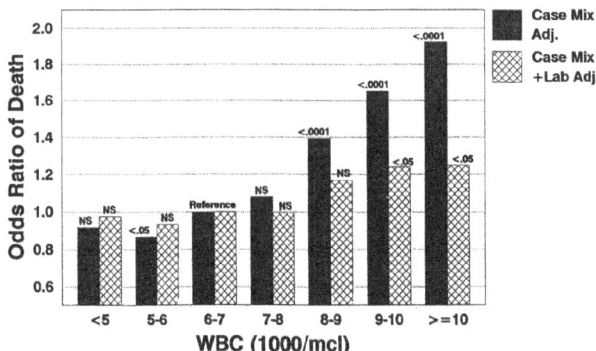

Fig. 16.   Risk profile for white blood count (WBC).

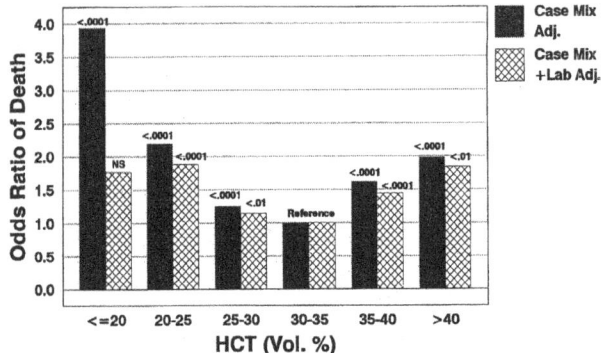

Fig. 17.   Risk profile for hematocrit.

Table 3. 1991 mortality analysis additional laboratory variables logistic regression models[a]

Laboratory variables	N	β	Odds ratio	χ^2	p
Aluminum (mcg/dl)	13,604	0.00607	1.006	57.47	0.0001
Calcium ion. (mg/dl)	5,200	−0.24060	0.786	10.26	0.0014
CA * P	16,322	−0.02470	0.976	2.20	NS
Magnesium (meq/l)	2,955	0.11740	1.125	0.85	NS
PTH intact (pg/ml)	8,245	−0.00009	1.000	0.61	NS
TIBC (mcg/dl)	14,741	−0.00047	1.000	0.41	NS
PTH–C term. (pg/ml)	3,846	0.00001	1.000	0.16	NS

[a] Adjusted for case mix and lab variables.

hematocrit exceeds 35 vol%. We wish to emphasize this U-shaped profile, however, because it is the second time we have observed it using different data sets. We believe it fair to say, therefore, that hematocrits above 35 vol% cannot be shown to improve the death risk profile of dialysis patients.

Non-routine laboratory variables

Table 3 shows the results of adding selected laboratory values, one at a time, to the Base Statistical Model which adjusts for both case mix and laboratory variables. The number of observations, regression coefficient (β), odds ratio and χ^2 statistic with its associated 'p' value are shown. Both serum aluminum concentration and ionized calcium were significantly associated with death risk. Calcium x phosphorous product, magnesium concentration, intact PTH, C-terminal PTH, and iron binding capacity were not. The finding of 'no significant association' does *not* mean that the variable is unimportant. For example, transferrin was adjusted for both albumin and creatinine in this analysis. Without such adjustment it may well have been a significant risk factor. The finding of significance by these analyses, therefore, implies that

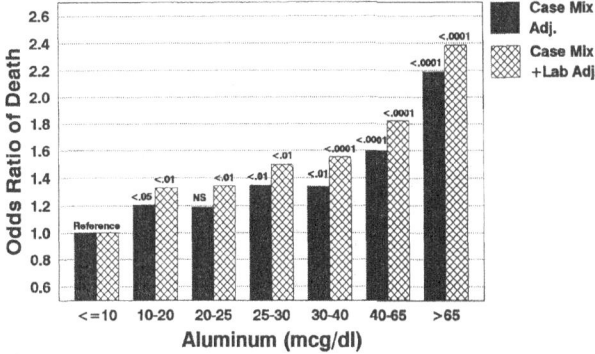

Fig. 18. Risk profile for unstimulated serum aluminum concentration.

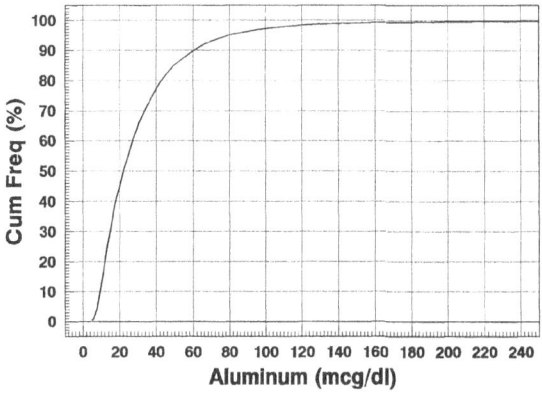

Fig. 19. Cumulative relative frequency histogram for unstimulated serum aluminum concentration.

additional information is not gained from their inclusion in the base statistical model.

Figure 18 shows the risk profile for serum aluminum (unstimulated) concentration. Patients with values ≤ 10 mcg/dl were selected as the reference group. The odds of death increases progressively in both case mix and case mix plus lab adjusted models as aluminum increases. The finding of interest is that Odds$_{aluminum}$ increases at such low levels of unstimulated aluminum concentration – anything over 10 mcg/dl. This finding supports previous analyses in which survivorship (i.e., survival curves) were determined as a function of initial serum aluminum concentration [6] suggested reduced survival as aluminum increases.

Figure 19 shows the cumulative relative frequency distribution for serum aluminum concentration. Approximately 90% of values exceeded 10 mcg/dl and 55% exceeded 20 mcg/dl. Hence, a large fraction of our dialysis patients continue to bear a substantial death risk burden associated with high serum aluminum concentration.

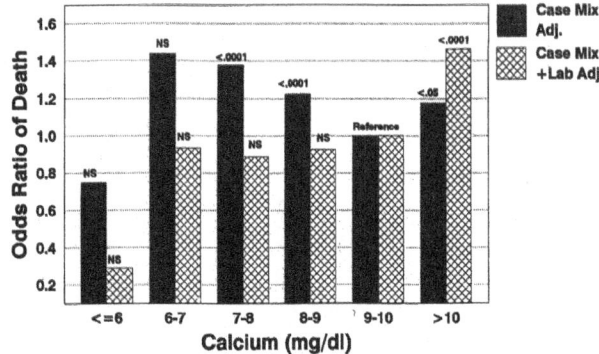

Fig. 20.   Risk profile for serum calcium concentration. Please compare to Fig. 21.

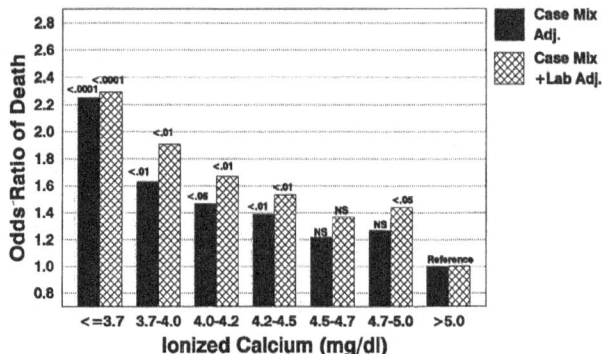

Fig. 21.   Risk profile for ionized serum calcium concentration. Please compare to Fig. 20.

Figures 20 and 21 show death risk profiles for serum calcium and ionized calcium concentration respectively. The difference is interesting. Serum calcium has never produced a dramatic risk profile in our analyses [1]. This is our first attempt at determining risk profile as a function of ionized calcium concentration. The odds of death increase progressively as ionized calcium falls. Hence, one should probably follow ionized rather than total serum calcium concentration in our patients.

Non-laboratory variables – the restricted sample

A separate database maintained on erythropoietin treated patients contains non-laboratory data which include height and periodic determinations of weight, systolic blood pressure, diastolic blood pressure, and transfusions. Nine thousand eighty (9, 080) patient records with complete data (all of the variables shown in Table 1 including both significant and non-significant variables, as well as determinations of height, weight, blood pressure, and so forth) were available for analysis. We transformed height and weight to percent ideal weight [7] and included all variables in the statistical model.

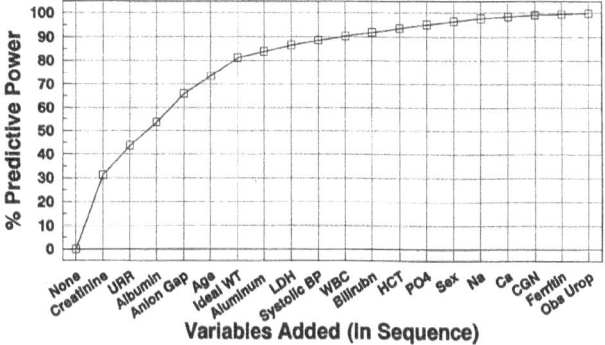

Variables Added (In Sequence)

Fig. 22. The fraction of final predictive power is shown as variables are added sequentially to a logistic model using a restricted sample of patients on which ideal weight and blood pressure measurements were available.

Table 4. Mortality analysis, 1991 data case mix & laboratory predictors[a] restricted sample

	Entry χ^2	Final model		
		Odds ratio	χ^2	p
Variables				
Creatinine (mg/dl)	356.3	0.851	132.3	0.0001
URR (%)	151.9	0.947	115.5	0.0001
Albumin (gm/dl)	122.2	0.367	78.3	0.0001
Anion gap	144.5	1.063	21.9	0.0001
Age (yrs)	92.1	1.031	132.1	0.0001
Ideal weight (%)	86.3	0.989	49.5	0.0001
Aluminum (mcg/dl)	37.3	1.006	37.9	0.0001
LDH (u/l)	35.6	1.004	28.2	0.0001
Systolic BP (mm Hg)	24.4	0.990	32.5	0.0001
WBC (1000/mcl)	23.2	1.070	18.1	0.0001
Bilirubin (mg/dl)	19.4	1.844	13.7	0.0002
HCT (%)	20.9	0.955	21.5	0.0001
Phosphorus (mg/dl)	18.0	1.140	27.1	0.0001
Sex (Ref = Male)	17.6	0.721	21.7	0.0001
Sodium (meq/l)	15.4	0.961	13.8	0.0002
Calcium (mg/dl)	10.1	1.148	10.0	0.0016
Glomerulonephritis	7.1	0.720	8.1	0.0043
Ferritin (ng/ml)	6.1	1.000	6.1	0.0137
Obs uropathy acq.	4.6	0.503	4.5	0.0341

[a] N = 9,080; Total model χ^2 = 1233.20; R^2 = 0.1535.

Figure 22 shows the sequenced selection of those variables into the model while Table 4 shows the entry χ^2 statistic, the odds ratio, the final model χ^2 and its associated p value. Creatinine, URR, and serum albumin concentration are again the first 3 variables added to the model while anion gap is the fourth. Age remains the 5th but there are now new 6th and 7th variables. Ideal weight (%) and aluminum concentration replace LDH and bilirubin. Thus, 7 variables

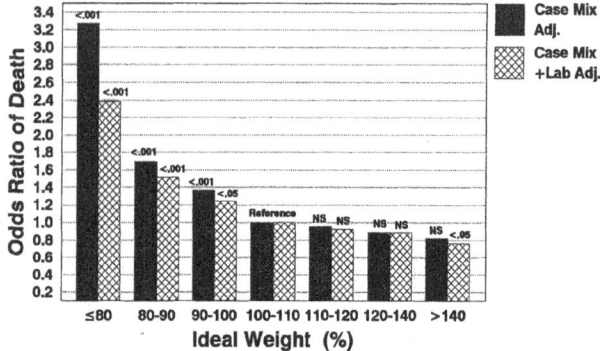

Fig. 23.   Risk profile for percent ideal weight.

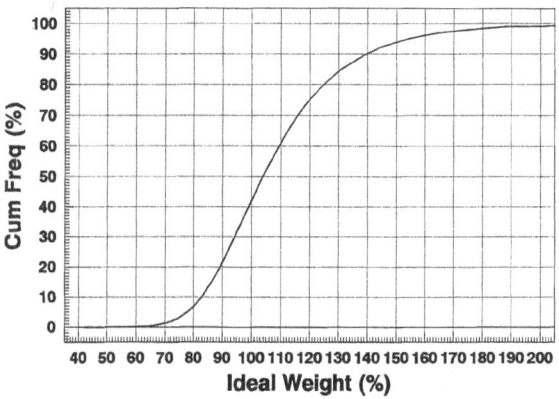

Fig. 24.   Cumulative relative frequency histogram of percent ideal weight.

account for about 83% of the final model predictive power. Adding LDH and systolic blood pressure account for another 5–6%.

Figure 23 shows the risk profile of ideal weight (%) adjusted for case mix only and for case mix and laboratory variables. Any value below 100% ideal weight is associated with increased odds of death in both models. Persons with ideal weight between 90% and 100% showed Odds$_{idealweight}$ of 1.2 to 1.4 times that of persons with ideal weight at or over 100%. Relative risk increases progressively as the fraction of ideal weight falls so that the odds of death exceeds 2.4 when patients' ideal weights are 80% or less.

Figure 24 shows the distribution of ideal weights in the 12, 495 patients on whom an ideal weight estimate was available. Approximately, 42% of patients had ideal weight which was < 100%. Approximately, 21% of patients had ideal weight which was < 90%.

Both systolic and diastolic blood pressure were associated with death risk. However, they were highly correlated and after adjustment for systolic pressure, diastolic pressure was no longer a significant death risk predictor. Figure 25 shows the risk profile for systolic blood pressure. The reference value was 120–135 mm Hg. Figure 26 shows the cumulative relative frequency distribu-

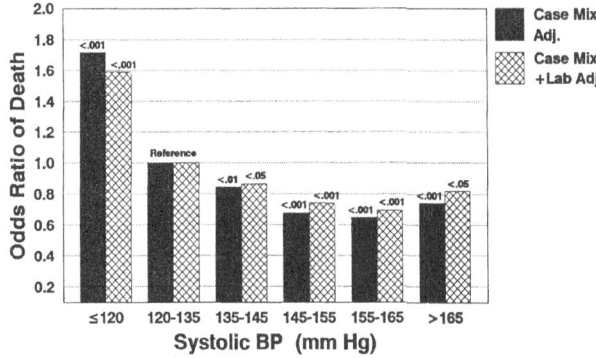

Fig. 25. Risk profile for systolic blood pressure.

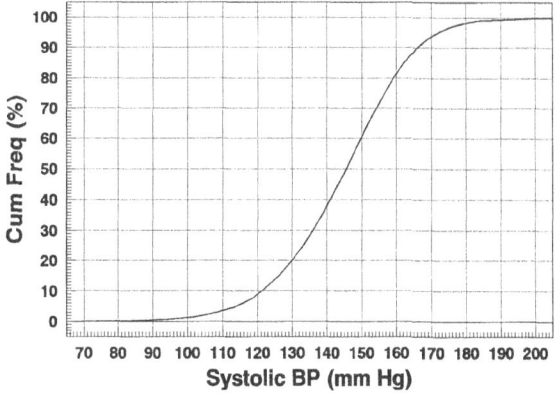

Fig. 26. Cumulative relative frequency histogram for pre-dialysis systolic blood pressure.

tion of systolic blood pressures on 16, 591 patients for whom these data were available. Approximately, 18% of patients had blood pressure exceeding 160 while slightly less than 10% had blood pressures of greatest risk which were ≤ 120 mm Hg.

Blood pressure was a moderately strong predictor of risk equivalent (say) to aluminum, LDH, and serum phosphorous. The orderly progression of risk upward as pressure falls seems reasonably convincing. The odds of death for patients was approximately 1.6 times the reference value when systolic pressure was ≤ 120 mm Hg. Furthermore, death risk fell progressively until pre-dialysis systolic pressure was in the range of 155–165 mm Hg. It increased slightly thereafter. The finding is counter-intuitive. It is interesting on two accounts. First, it does not change much with adjustment for laboratory values. Second, the level of lowest risk is at much higher blood pressure than we would have anticipated.

Afterthoughts

These analyses once again illustrate the critical importance of nutrition to the health of dialysis patients. New data are provided. The risk of lower than normal ideal weight reinforces other findings about albumin and creatinine concentrations [1, 2, 4, 5]. The clinical dynamics of anion gap which likely includes nutritional considerations deserves further investigation.

Four of the six variables contributing about 80% of the statistical predictive power suggested by Fig. 22 are related to the nutrition of patients – creatinine, albumin, anion gap, and percent of ideal weight. The other two are URR and age. Because we can do little about the age of patients, these analyses focus attention clearly on dialysis intensity (URR) and nutrition as the two areas of clinical endeavor particularly deserving of attention if the goal is to reduce mortal risk among our patients. Other maladies such as anemia, increased burdens of aluminum, liver disease, and so forth must not be neglected. But the combination of nutritional status and dialysis intensity appear to contribute most to mortal risk.

Sobering inferences emerge from contemplating data of these sorts, however. The R^2 statistic of these and other analyses are generally in the range of 0.14–0.20 [1, 2, 4]. While the probablistic associations are strong and must not be ignored, the finding suggests that measured variables explain only 20% or less of the death risk differences among patients. The National Cooperative Dialysis Study recruited highly selected patients and studied them in a highly controlled way [9]. Yet the measured variables explained only about 20% of the differences in the odds of failure between patients [9]. Even when other variables were added to those statistical analyses the maximum coefficient of determination was only about 30% [9]. Therefore, focusing solely on dialysis intensity, the nutritional status of patients, and the expanded list of death predictors such as liver disease, blood pressure, and the body burden of aluminum, may lead us to overlook systematic strategies of possible benefit to patients. The minds of those who study or deliver clinical care must be open to other potential strategies as well. This realization implies the continuing need for exploratory analyses which include expanded lists of empirically determined potential predictors of morbidity and mortality.

References

1. Lowrie EG, Lew NL. Death risk in hemodialysis patients: The predictive value of commonly measured variables and an evaluation of death rate differences between facilities. Am J Kid Dis 1990; 15 (5): 458–482.
2. Lowrie EG, Lew NL. Commonly measured laboratory variables in hemodialysis patients: relationships among them and to death risk. Seminars in Nephrology 1992; 12 (3): 276–283.
3. Hosmer DW, Lemeshow S. Applied logistic regression. J Wiley & Sons, New York, 1989.
4. Lowrie EG, Lew NL, Huang WH. Race and diabetes as death risk predictors in hemodialysis patients. Kidney Int 1992; 42 (Suppl 38): S22-S31.
5. Owen WF, Jr., Lew NL, Liu Y, Lowrie EG, Lazarus JM. Urea reduction ratio and serum albumin: mortality predictors for hemodialysis. Submitted to NEJM for publication, 1993.

6. Chazan JA, Lew NL, Lowrie EG. Increased serum aluminum. An independent risk factor for mortality in patients undergoing long-term hemodialysis. Arch Intern Med 1991; 151: 319–322.
7. 1983 Metropolitan Height and Weight Tables.
8. Lowrie EG, Laird NM, Henry RR. Protocol for the National Cooperative Dialysis Study. Kidney Int 1983; 23 (Suppl 13): S11-S18.
9. Laird NM, Berkey CS, Lowrie EG. Modeling success or failure of dialysis therapy: the National Cooperative Dialysis Study. Kidney Int 1983; 23 (Suppl 13): S101-S106.

CHAPTER 14

Short hemodialysis: big trouble in a small package

ROBERT H. BARTH

Introduction

One of the characteristic features of the brief three-decade history of hemodialysis has been the progressive decline of the duration of individual treatment sessions. For some – including many patients – this has represented
a clear and relentless march forward in the quality and effectiveness of our
therapeutic technique. A scant decade ago, the questions being asked about
short dialysis reflected the feeling that only technological obstacles blocked
the almost unlimited shortening of treatment time [1, 2]. One of the topics
at a symposium like this one bore the title '2-h dialysis: A realistic goal?'
[3], and a 1988 editorial asking 'Are there limitations to shortening dialysis
treatment?' [4] did not answer in the affirmative.

Skeptical voices are, however, increasingly heard, and the question now
being asked about short dialysis is quite a different one. Since the startling
mortality figures for the United States End Stage Renal Disease program
became known in 1989 [5] suspicion – and evidence – has accumulated that
the shortening of dialysis sessions which took place throughout the 1980s
in this country was at least partially responsible. [6, 7] Nevertheless, short
sessions remain popular, and the questions need asking yet again: What is the
evidence linking too short dialysis with higher mortality, and how short *is* too
short?

Setting the stage

In order for short dialysis to have had such widespread adoption, three factors
were necessary: technical feasibility, economic incentives, and a means of
medical/scientific rationalization and justification.

The first prerequisite to technical viability was the demonstration that
short dialysis could in fact be done without serious deterioration in patient
wellbeing. In 1973, the standard for dialysis was still sessions of eight hours

143

E. A. Friedman (ed.), Death on Hemodialysis, 143–157.
© 1994 *Kluwer Academic Publishers.*

Table 1. Short dialysis: clinical studies

Authors	Date	N	Dialyzer		Mode[b]	K (ml/min)	V (l)	t (h)	Kt/V[c]	Followup (mo)
			N	Membrane[a]						
[9]	1975	101	1	Ce	HD			3.5–4.0	0.68–078	≤ 24
[10]	1976	12	2	Ce	HD			4.47	1.10	12–18
[11]	1976	13	2	Ce	HD	163		3.00	0.73	2
[12]	1981	2	2	PA	HF	263	45.4[d]	2.00	0.70	18
[13]	1983	16	1	PAN	HDF	305		2.17	0.99	3
[1]	1984	4	2	CA	HDF	407	47.4[d]	1.92	0.99	0.5
[2]	1985	25	2	Ce	HD	436	36.4[d]	2.00	1.44	12
[14]	1986	112	1	CA	HED	265	36.7[d]	2.88	1.25	10
[15]	1992	56	1	PS	HFD	285	41.5	2.45	1.01	6–30

[a] CA = cellulose acetate; Ce = cellulose; PA = polyamide; PS = polysulfone; PAN = polyacrylonitrile.
[b] HD = hemodiafiltration; HED = high-efficiency hemodialysis; HF = hemofiltration; HFD = flux hemodialysis
[c] Best estimate from data provided.
[d] Calculated from 0.55 × body weight.

or more with the Kiil parallel-plate dialyzer. Vincenzo Cambi, in Parma, Italy, was the first to experiment with the drastically shortened schedule of 10.5 to 12 hours per week, using disposable cellulose dialyzers [8, 9]. The Parma group was able to demonstrate acceptable results, despite higher levels of blood urea, and by the end of the 1970s disposable dialyzers and four to five hour treatments were the rule. Reasoning that increased dialysis membrane surface area would allow solute removal in shorter times, a number of groups sought "ultrashort" times by the use of several dialyzers in series or parallel, often using hemofiltration or hemodiafiltration to increase middle-molecule clearance (Table 1). By the mid-eighties treatment times of less than three hours per session had been shown to be feasible, if not always practical, given the complexity of the systems involved.

There were problems with intradialytic symptoms, however, and the headaches, nausea, and hemodynamic instability were at first ascribed to dysequilibrium phenomena or 'unphysiology' [15] which would have sharply limited the wide applicability of high-clearance techniques. Later it became clear that the culprit was in fact the acetate ion in the dialysate, and the increasing availability of practical dialysis delivery systems using bicarbonate dialysate may have been the development which most facilitated mass application of rapid dialysis methods [14]. The combination of high-sodium, bicarbonate dialysate, volumetric ultrafiltration, and large surface area dialyzers with highly permeable membranes seem to bring safe three-hour treatments within reach of any dialysis unit [15] although costs remained disconcertingly high.

Mere availability of methods does not make for mass acceptance, but short treatments fitted the needs of providers and patients alike. Shrinking Medicare reimbursement rates, which fell throughout the 'eighties in both in real and inflated dollars provided the economic incentive to shorten individual treatments and maximize the profitability of available resources [6] Held and colleagues [16], studying the relationships between funding and treatment duration, found that the degree of reduction of time practiced in dialysis units after the Medicare reimbursement cuts of 1983 was related to the extent of decreased funding in each unit, and that the shortest treatments were received by patients in for-profit units. Manufacturers of dialyzers and delivery systems caught the temper of the times with marketing campaigns based on their products' urea clearance and ability to deliver shortened dialysis [17]. Patients cheerfully accepted any new approach which could reduce their time spent fettered to a dialysis machine.

Nonetheless, for years it had been well known that insufficient dialysis leads to serious morbidity and mortality, so the mere availability of 'high-efficiency' techniques and the largely short-term feasibility studies listed in Table 1 would not have been enough, even in the political/economic context of the 'eighties, to drive wide adoption of short treatment times. Arbitrary limitation of dialysis treatment without some scientific justification and ability to mathematically define an indicated 'dose' would have been intellectually and ethically suspect. By mid-decade, however, the mathematical tools were at hand. The National Cooperative Dialysis Study (NCDS) had been completed, and its findings published in 1983, and, despite the secondary conclusion that decreased dialysis time independently worsened morbidity [18], measurement of blood urea had been established as the sole yardstick for dialysis therapy. In 1985, analyzing further the data from the NCDS, Gotch and Sargent [19] introduced the 'dialysis index' or Kt/V – the product of dialyzer urea clearance and treatment duration normalized to the patient's volume of distribution for urea – as the fundamental tool for prescribing and monitoring hemodialysis, and defined a value for this index which there was 'no apparent clinical value' in exceeding. The concept of a mathematically definable dialysis dose was thus confirmed, the measuring instrument – urea modeling – was provided and, of greatest importance, a reciprocal relationship between urea clearance and time was established. Dialyzer manufacturers were quick to understand and exploit the equation 'More Efficient Urea Removal = Shorter Time = Greater Profitability'. Urea modeling was invoked – although perhaps not frequently practiced – as justification for shortening treatments throughout the United States [20].

The United States: Cutting close to the dialytic bone

The extent to which shortened time has been embraced in the United States is suggested by Table 2, which shows the results of two studies of dialysis prescription in large populations – the 237 units of the National Medical Care proprietary dialysis chain [21], and a cohort of 3,757 patients starting dialysis in 1986–87, followed by the United States Renal Data System [22]. As can be seen, about 60% of the patients receive 3.5 hours or less per treatment.

Table 2. Dialysis time in two large studies in the United States

	Patients	Weekly dialysis time		
		< 9 hr	9–10.5 hr[a]	> 10.5 hr
National Medical Care [21]	19746	40%	18%	42%
USRDS 1986–87 incident cohort [22]	3757	17%	52%	31%

[a] USRDS data are for 9–11 hr.

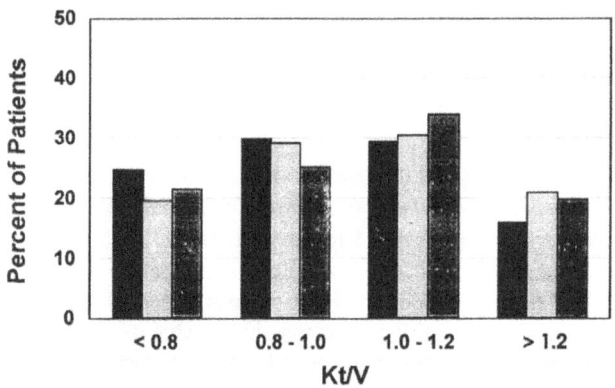

Fig. 1.   Dialysis 'dose' (Kt/V) received by patients in three large surveys. About 50% of patients in each group received treatments with Kt/V < 1.0, considered inadequate therapy. ■ Gotch *et al.* [26], 101 patients; ☐, Delmez *et al.* [23], 617 patients; ▨, USRDS [22], 3096 patients.

In fact, the median weekly treatment time for the USRDS patients was 9.0 hours, indicating that fully one-half were treated for 3 hours or less. [22] That these figures are representative of US practice is confirmed by the findings of the St. Louis Nephrology Study Group [23], which examined hemodialysis delivery for 617 patients in 16 outpatient units in metropolitan St. Louis and found a mean treatment length of 3.2 ± 0.4 hours. Infatuation with short time appears to be primarily a United States phenomenon; USRDS data for European diaylsis prescriptions shows a mean weekly treatment time of 12.1 hours and a median of 11.3 hour [22], and similar information showing mean treatment lengths of well over 4 hours is available from Australia [24] and Japan [25].

One might expect that with reliance on mathematical prescription an adequate 'dose' would be maintained by increasing dialyzer efficiency as time

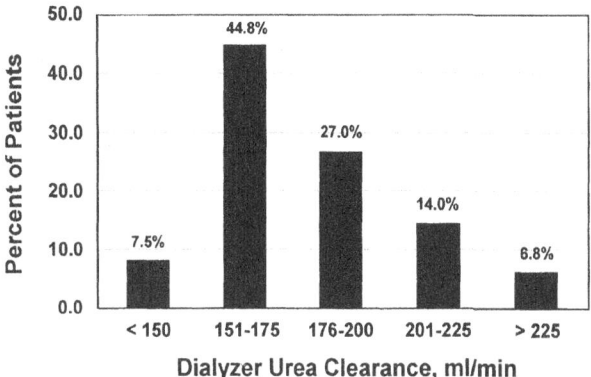

Fig. 2. Prescribed dialyzer urea clearance in 3096 U.S. patients. The clearances are determined from manufacturer-supplied data. The overall mean is 181.5 ml/min. (From [22]).

is cut, but this does not seem to be the case. Even by the original standards for dialysis adequacy developed in the Gotch analysis of the NCDS – that is, a value of Kt/V of 1.0 or more – US dialysis seems deficient. Figure 1 shows the results of three surveys of dialysis prescription in relatively random population [22, 23, 26]. In each study, about one-half of the patients receive less than what is considered by rather conservative standards to be a minimum dose of dialysis. In fact, there is little evidence that prescription of shorter time is accompanied by use of larger, more efficient dialyzers. Figure 2, from the USRDS data [22], shows prescribed urea clearances in 3096 patients. A glance at Table 1 quickly reveals that the clearances used in the dialysis series of the 1980's which serve as the prototypes for shortening of dialysis are far higher than the clearances actually used in practice, even though treatment times in the highly controlled investigative series are quite similar to times used in the outpatient units surveyed above. In addition, the USRDS clearance data are based on manufacturers' specifications, probably the least reliable source (see below), and so the degree of underdelivery of dialysis demonstrated by these figures may be an underestimate.

Compounding these problems of inadequate dialysis is the real question of what the minimum 'dose' should be. In the reasoning which underlies urea modeling, the blood urea concentration serves as a surrogate marker for larger, presumably toxic products of protein metabolism. As time is shortened and clearance (one hopes) is increased, the relationship of urea and these larger molecules may well change, thereby changing the significance of urea concentrations [20] As the rate of dialytic removal increases, the importance of membrane resistance to diffusion of urea and larger molecules from the

Table 3. Kt/V and patient survival on hemodialysis

Unit	N	Kt/V	Survival			
			1 year	2 year	5 year	10 year
USRDS 1991 [37]	34058	0.8?	78%	61%	38%	25%
Taiwan # 1 [32]	505	1.5		78%		
Taiwan # 2 [32]	227	1.8		89%		
Tassin, FR [36]	445	1.7			87%	75%
Vanderbilt [35][a]	120	0.8	77%			
	120	0.9	82%			
	120	1.0	84%			
	120	1.2	91%			

[a] Vanderbilt data are for consecutive years.

intracellular space – a far less important consideration at the low removal rates used in the NCDS – becomes more and more significant [27, 28]. In short, the model becomes less valid, and the meaning of a given Kt/V changes. For these reasons, higher minimum values of Kt/V than 1.0 have been recommended on purely theoretical grounds for short hemodialysis [29].

Further, both a reexamination of the NCDS data and Gotch's analysis [30, 31], and clinical studies of the relationship of urea removal and patient outcome [32–36] indicate that both morbidity and mortality are improved by dialysis with a Kt/V of 1.2 or more, and it may be reasonable to believe that optimal dialysis requires a Kt/V as high as 1.4 [31]. Table 3 shows the effect of higher levels of Kt/V on mortality, with USRDS data shown for comparison. While these studies largely lack simultaneous controls, the data are nonetheless striking, and strongly suggest an effect of increasing Kt/V well beyond even 1.2. In this light, the US statistics on prescribed Kt/V appear even more grim.

Shortness and Death

The grimmest of all US hemodialysis statistics is, of course, the remarkably high gross mortality which first came to public attention in 1989 [5]. The serious underdelivery of dialysis described in the preceding paragraphs might suffice to explain this, but the question which concerns us here is the role of short time both in accounting for the underdialysis and in independently affecting mortality.

The earliest epidemiological hint that shortening of dialysis might be related to deterioration of patient outcome came from the European Dialysis and Transplant Association, which had long been more effective at data collection than any similar organization in the United States. At the 1982 meeting, as part of the yearly report, it was revealed that "the proportion of deaths in the Federal Republic of Germany was twice as high in short dialysis ... and that of deaths due to myocardial infarction was higher in males on short dialysis" [37]. This theme of the cardiovascular dangers of short dialysis has been expanded upon by Wizemann and Kramer [38], who themselves were pioneers of 'ultrashort' treatment, but who later abandoned the technique because of high cardiovascular morbidity. Control of extracellular fluid volume is certainly more difficult in many patients treated with three-hour or shorter dialyses, and the resultant hypertension and extensive use of antihypertensive medication may contribute markedly to the atherosclerotic and cardiac complications of end-stage renal disease [39]. The remarkable survival statistics shown in shown in Table 3 from the Centre de rein artificiel at Tassin, France, where eight-hour dialyses are still the rule, have been ascribed to the scrupulous control of hypertension with minimal use of drugs achieved by the long dialysis sessions [36, 39]. A compelling syllogism results: in the United States, where short dialysis is the rule, hypertension in dialysis patients is poorly controlled [40]; hypertension is a major predictor of morbidity and mortality in dialysis patients [36, 39, 41]. Can one escape the conclusion that short dialysis increases mortality?

The relationship between dialysis treatment duration and mortality has been investigated directly, with disturbing results. Figure 3 shows the effect of treatment time on mortality risk for 600 randomly chosen patients in 36 dialysis units across the United States [42] (A), and for 12,099 patients in 237 National Medical Care facilities reported by Lowrie and Lew [21](B). In both cases mortality increases significantly as treatment time is reduced. These data are impossible to ignore; shorter dialysis is incontrovertibly related to higher mortality.

One interpretation of this finding, which is frequently cited by defenders of short treatment regimens [26, 29], is that short time is not the culprit – it is instead the ill-advised reduction of treatment duration without sufficient monitoring and increase of dialyzer efficiency. On the surface, this sounds eminently reasonable; why, then, have such adjustments apparently not taken place on such a vast scale in the US? Are American nephrologists ignorant, venal, or sadistic?

Lies, damned lies, and dialyzer clearance data

Since system-wide evildoing on the part of nephrologists is unlikely to be the cause of the widespread inadequacy that now characterizes US hemodialysis prescriptions, an examination of the prescription process and its possibilities is in order. Leaving aside for the moment discussions of the validity of urea kinetic modeling itself [20], one may accept as a working definition of adequacy of dialysis the maintenance of a Kt/V greater than 1.20. This is a relatively conservative position, and one, I think, that would draw little argument from most proponents of urea monitoring. Our task will be to understand what kind and degree of compensation is necessary when reducing dialysis time to three hours or less.

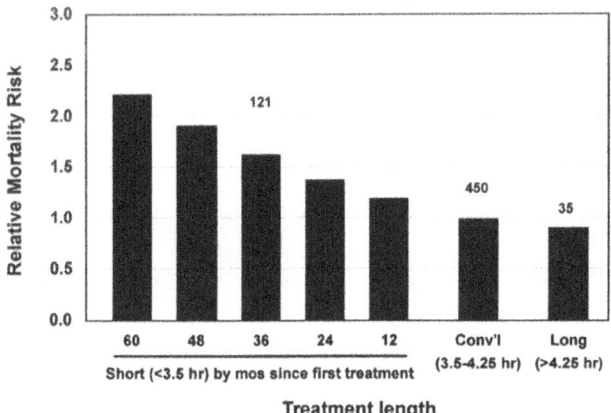

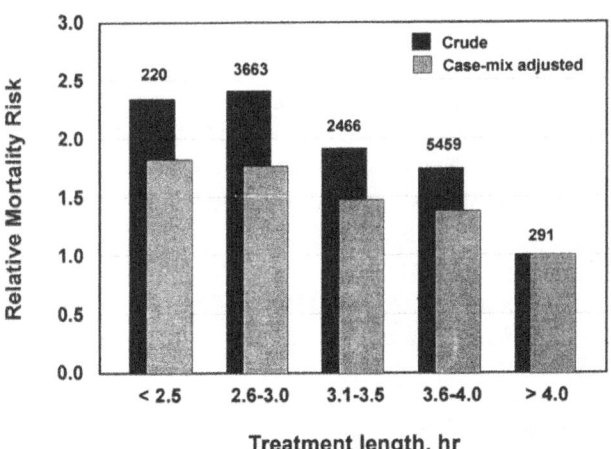

Fig. 3. Relative mortality risk vs. dialysis treatment length. (a) 600 patients studied by Held *et al.* show higher mortality risk with treatment times less than 3.5 hours, and increasing risk with more months of exposure [42]; (b) National Medical Care patients show increasing mortality risk with each decrement of treatment time from greater than 4.0 to less than 2.5 hours [21]. Numbers above bars are patients at risk.

To maintain Kt/V at a given level when t is reduced, one has clearly few options. V is a fixed characteristic of the patient, closely related to total body water, and is not amenable to therapeutic manipulation, leaving only K, the dialyzer urea clearance, available for adjustment. This adjustment in K normally takes place in one of two ways, by increasing blood flow rate or by changing the dialyzer itself to one with a higher surface area, a more permeable membrane, or both. Since there is no increase in cost and no apparent side effects from increasing blood flow rate [43, 44], and clearance is significantly increased by raising blood flow rate to 400 ml/min with virtually every dialyzer in use today [45], it remains unclear why anyone is dialyzed at less than the maximum flow rate obtainable through their vascular access, certainly at least 400 ml/min if possible. Nevertheless, the USRDS has found that in a group of more than 4,000 randomly chosen patients beginning dialysis in 1986–87 the median blood flow rate used was 250 ml/min [46].

Let us assume, however, a blood flow of 400 ml/min. What dialyzer urea clearance is necessary to adequately treat in three hours or less? The answer depends, of course, on the size of the patient and the consequent value of V. A frequently used approximation of V is 55% of body weight, which gives a value of 38.5 liters for a 70 kg person. In fact, mean kinetically-derived values of V for large populations are in this range – Dumler *et al* [15] reported a value of 41.5 liters for their 56 patients on short high-flux dialysis, and in 127 dialyses monitored with direct quantification of dialysate urea [47, 48], we have found a mean V of 36.9 liters.

Figure 4 presents the relationships between K, t and V (expressed as body weight) in graphic form for a dialysis which will provide Kt/V = 1.2. Inspection of the graph reveals that for a 3-hour dialysis, a 70-kg patient would require a dialyzer urea clearance of 276 ml/min, and for a 2.5-hour dialysis, 336 ml/min would be necessary. It is now important to know whether these are realistic clearances, obtainable with currently available equipment. Table 4 shows dialyzer clearances obtained by measurement of the urea in the entire volume of spent dialysate, an extremely accurate measure of effective clearance. The values in the table have been corrected upward to compensate for the effect of access recirculation, measured in all cases, which was 11.4 ± 7.9 % (mean ± SD). No measured clearance was higher than 300 ml/min. The larger surface-area high-efficiency dialyzers, like the F–60, F–80 and CA210 were able to achieve 240–260 ml/min, but it is unlikely that much higher values can be reached with a single dialyzer.

The situation is now clear. With the best available dialyzer, the highest blood and dialysate flows, and a well-functioning access, a patient weighing 70-kg or less *might* achieve a Kt/V of 1.2 in 3 hours. In 2.5 hours it is not possible with currently available equipment. But patients are not being dialyzed with the largest dialyzers and the highest blood flows – looking again at the USRDS 1986–87 cohort, we find that only 3% were dialyzed with high-flux membranes [46]. The second part of Table 4 shows conventional dialyzer clearances at blood flows of 330–350 ml/min. The best dialyzer

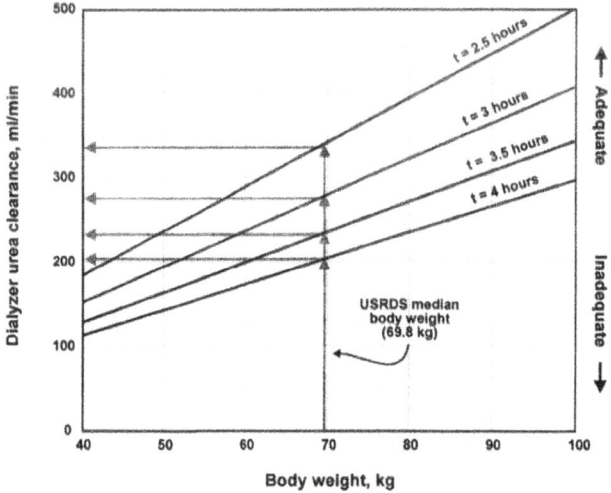

Fig. 4.   Dialyzer urea clearance required to provide Kt/V = 1.2 at various treatment lengths. Any clearance above the time line for a given body weight will provide Kt/v = 1.2. Thus, for a patient weighing 69.8 kg, a clearance of 202 ml/min for 4 hours or 336 ml/min for 2.5 hours will provide Kt/V = 1.2. A blood flow rate of 400 ml/min and access recirculation of 10% are assumed.

approaches, but does not reach, 200 ml/min; the overall mean clearance value is 176 ml/min, not much different from the mean prescribed clearance of 182 ml/min for the USRDS patients.

But prescribed clearances are often based on manufacturer-supplied data, which, because they are often based on so-called *in vitro* measurements using aqueous solutions of urea, because they are frequently extrapolated from measurements made at low dialysate and blood flow rates, and because they take no account of clearance losses from intradialytic blood clotting, recirculation, and the like, almost always grossly overestimate dialyzer performance. Prescriptions are formulated on the basis of inflated clearance values which have little basis in reality, and dangerously inadequate treatments result [49]. Add to this the effects of erythropoietin-stimulated hematocrits [50], access recirculation [51], and the various forms of temporal cornercutting that often occur in a busy dialysis unit, and it is not surprising that, to paraphrase LeFebvre *et al* [52]. patients do not get what the physician *thinks* she prescribes.

Returning to the question, how short is too short, we have seen that for most patients, three hours is too short even with high-flux dialyzers. With the largest conventional dialyzers, as shown in Fig. 5, only a patient weighing

Table 4. Dialyzer urea clearances by total dialysate collection and from manufacturers' data

Dialyzer	Manufac-turer	Mem-brane[a]	N	Blood flow ml/min	K by DQU ml/min	K from manuf. ml/min
High-flux:						
CA–210	Baxter	CA	7	500	253	322
Duoflux	Cordis-Dow	CA	7	486	183	252
F–60	Fresenius	PS	5	443	256	290
F–80M	Fresenius	PS	5	390	239	281
Filtral 12	Hospal	SPAN	23	544	196	244
Filtral 16	Hospal	SPAN	27	538	230	281
Total high-flux						
Conventional:						
CA–90	Baxter	CA	7	311	163	210
CD–4000	Cordis-Dow	CA	5	350	148	187
135sce	Cordis-Dow	SCE	10	338	198	229
155sec	Cordis-Dow	SCE	3	350	177	234
F–5	Fresenius	PS	6	338	177	231
Total conventional			31	335	176	219

[a] CA = cellulose acetate; PS = polysulfone; SCE = saponified cellulose ester; SPAN = sulfonated polyacrylonitrile

less than 52 kg can be dialyzed in three hours with a Kt/V of 1.2 or more. A 70 kg patient cannot receive adequate dialysis in less than four hours, and a patient weighing 90 kg needs five hours. Some leeway is afforded by residual renal function, and it is probably for that reason that patients do as well as they do on short dialysis, since 1 or 2 ml/min of native glomerular filtration rate is the equivalent of 20–40 ml/min extra dialyzer clearance, considering only urea. As the residual renal function disappears, however, trouble will ensue for most patients on short dialysis the way it is performed in the United States.

Trying to brighten a bleak landscape

A few conclusions can be drawn:

– *Acceptable dialysis can be delivered in three hours or less, but only under optimal conditions,* such as low body weight, very high dialyzer urea clearance, and low access recirculation. Practically speaking, such conditions almost never obtain in the United States.

– *With most of the dialyzers in use in the United States, adequate dialysis cannot be delivered in three hours.* Most conventional dialyzers are incapable of adequately dialyzing a 70 kg patient in less than four hours, and many high-flux dialyzers cannot do it in three hours, even if anyone

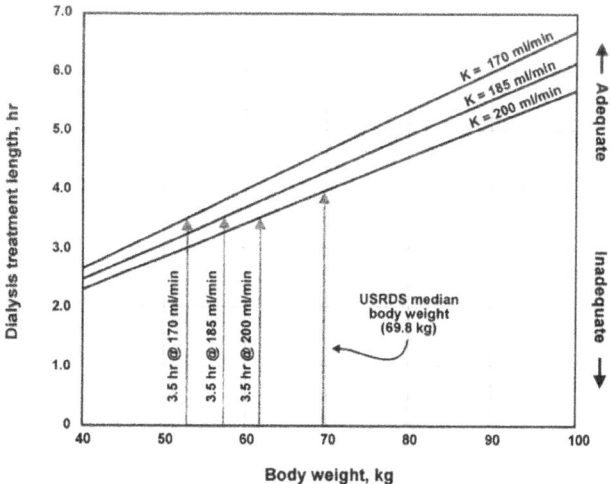

Fig. 5.   Time required to provide Kt/V = 1.2 at various dialyzer clearances. Shown are the maximum body weights for achieving the desired Kt/V in 3.5 hours. With a dialyzer which clears urea at 185 ml/min, the largest patient who will receive adequate dialysis in 3.5 hours weighs 57 kg. A 70-kg patient requires 4 hours with a 200 ml/min dialyzer, 4.6 hours with one which clears at 170 ml/min. A blood flow rate of 350 ml/min and access recirculation of 5% are assumed.

used them. The exceptions, of course, are very small patients and those who have significant residual renal function.

– *Most of the dialysis prescribed in the United States is inadequate.* Available data indicate that most dialyses do not achieve a Kt/V of 1.0, let alone the more ambitious value of 1.2. Prescriptions, when they are based on anything other than custom, are frequently founded on erroneous, inflated dialyzer clearances supplied by manufacturers.

– *Short (3 hour or less) dialysis should only be used for patients who have significant residual renal function.*

Evidence can be found at every turn of the serious underdelivery of dialysis in the United States, and it is our patients who pay the piper. More careful monitoring, more use of Urea Reduction Ratios, and use of higher blood and dialysate flows all may help, but when all is said and done, the only solution to underdialysis is more dialysis. There are only two ways to accomplish that – bigger, more efficient dialyzers and longer time. There is demonstrable resistance to both in the United States, partly for understandable economic reasons, perhaps partly because of infatuation with the idea that shorter time is a kind of progress, the victory of technology over the forces of darkness, and partly because to many nephrologists, dialysis and dialysis patients seem an annoyance, whose presence is best minimized. For most people on dialysis, who are the reason we pursue these issues, Kt/V and urea modeling and adequacy are vague and distant concepts, with little or no force in their lives; they know only that an extra hour free of needles and machinery is a gift, not easily foregone. It is our responsibility as nephrologists not only to shepherd their hematocrits, but also to be their guide and advocate in the political minefield that American medicine may become, and we had better be clear about our goals. Optimal therapy, not adequate therapy, should be that goal, and we need to leave behind the dialytic philosophy of the bare minimum.

References

1. Von Albertini B, Miller JH, Gardner PW, Shinaberger JH. High-flux hemodiafiltration: Under six hours/week treatment. Trans ASAIO 1984; 30: 227–231.
2. Rotellar E, Martinez E, Samsó JM, et al. Why dialyze more than 6 hours a week? Trans ASAIO 1985; 31: 538–545.
3. Cambi V, Arisi L, David S, Bono F, Gardini G. 2-h dialysis: A realistic goal? Contrib Nephrol 1985; 44: 40–48.
4. Collins AJ, Keshaviah PR. Are there limitations to shortening dialysis treatment? Trans ASAIO 1988; 34: 1–5.
5. Hull AR, Parker TF. Introduction and summary: Proceedings from the Morbidity, Mortality and Prescription of Dialysis Symposium, Dallas TX, September 15 to 17, 1989. Am J Kidney Dis 1990; 15: 375–383.
6. Berger EE, Lowrie EG. Mortality and the length of dialysis. JAMA 1991; 265: 909–910.
7. Shaldon S, Koch KM. Survival and adequacy in long-term hemodialysis. Nephron 1991; 59: 353–357.
8. Cambi V, Arisi L, Buzio C, Rossi E, Savazzi G, Migone L. Intensive utilisation of a dialysis unit. Proc Eur Dial Transplant Assoc 1973; 10: 342–348.
9. Cambi V, Savazzi G, Arisi L, et al. Short dialysis schedules (SDS) – finally ready to become routine? Proc Eur Dial Transplant Assoc 1975; 11: 112–120.
10. Shaldon S, Florence P, Fontanier P, Polito C, Mion C. Comparison of two strategies for short dialysis using 1 m^2 and 2 m^2 surface area dialysers. Proc Eur Dial Transplant Assoc 1976; 12: 596–605.
11. Ben Ari J, Oren A, Berlyne GM. Short duration-high area regular dialysis using two UF 2 coils in series. Nephron 1976; 16: 74–79.
12. Shaldon S, Beau MC, Deschodt G, Mion C. Mixed hemofiltration (MHF): 18 months treatment with ultrashort treatment time. Trans ASAIO 1981; 27: 610–612.
13. Cioni L, Palmarini N, Pilone N, Rindi P. Hemodiafiltration: Better efficiency with respect to hemodialysis and hemofiltration. Blood Purif 1984; 2: 30–35.
14. Keshaviah P, Collins A. Rapid high-efficiency bicarbonate hemodialysis. Trans ASAIO 1986; 32: 17–23.
15. Kjellstrand CM, Rosa AA, Shideman JR, Rodrigo F, Davin T, Lynch RE. Optimal dialysis frequency and duration: the "unphysiology hypothesis". Kidney Int 1978; Suppl 8: S120–124.
16. Held PJ, García J, Pauly MV, Cahn MA. Price of dialysis, unit staffing, and length of dialysis treatments. Am J Kidney Dis 1990; 15: 441–450.
17. Held PJ, García J, Pauly MV, Cahn MA. Travenol systems to reduce treatment time. Travenol Laboratories, Inc., Deerfield IL, 1986.
18. Harter HR. Review of significant findings from the National Cooperative Dialysis Study and recommendations. Kidney Int 1983; 23 (Supp 13): S107–S112.

19. Gotch FA, Sargent JA. A mechanistic analysis of the National Cooperative Dialysis Study (NCDS). Kidney Int 1985; 28: 526–534.
20. Barth RHJ. Dialysis by the numbers: The false promise of Kt/V. Sem Dial 1989; 2: 207–212.
21. Lowrie EG, Lew NL. Death risk in hemodialysis patients: The predictive value of commonly measured variables and an evaluation of death rate differences between facilities. Am J Kidney Dis 1990; 15: 458–482.
22. US Renal Data System. USRDS 1992 Annual Report. The National Institutes of Health, National Institute of Diabetes and Digestive and Kidney Diseases, Bethesda MD, 1992.
23. Delmez JA, Windus DW, The St. Louis Nephrology Study Group. Hemodialysis prescription and delivery in a metropolitan community. Kidney Int 1992; 41: 1023–1028.
24. Disney APS. Prescription and practice of dialysis in Australia, 1988. Am J Kidney Dis 1990; 15: 494–499.
25. Iseki K, Kawazoe N, Osawa A, Fukiyama K. Survival analysis of dialysis patients in Okinawa, Japan (1971–1990). Kidney Int 1993; 43: 404–409.
26. Gotch FA, Yarian S, Keen M. A kinetic survey of US hemodialysis prescriptions. Am J Kidney Dis 1990; 15: 511–515.
27. Stiller S, Mann H. Ultra-short dialysis and internal physiologic resistance. Trans ASAIO 1987; 33: 754–757.
28. Lopot F. Is urea kinetic modelling an appropriate tool for guiding ultrashort highflux dialysis therapy? Nephrol Dial Transplant 1991; Suppl 3: 86–87.
29. Von Albertini B, Bosch JP. Short hemodialysis. Am J Nephrol 1991; 11: 169–173.
30. Keshaviah P, Collins A. A re-appraisal of the National Cooperative Dialysis Study (NCDS). Kidney Int 1988; 33: 227.
31. Hakim RM, Depner TA, Parker TF. Adequacy of hemodialysis. Am J Kidney Dis 1992; 20: 107–123.
32. Shen F-H, Hsu K-T. Lower mortality and morbidity associated with higher Kt/V in hemodialysis patients. J Am Soc Nephrol 1990; 1: 377.
33. Collins A, Liao M, Umen A, Hanson G, Keshaviah P. High-efficiency bicarbonate hemodialysis has a lower risk of death than standard acetate dialysis. J Am Soc Nephrol 1991; 2: 318.
34. Collins A, Liao M, Umen A, Hanson G, Keshaviah P. Diabetic hemodialysis patients treated with a high Kt/V have a lower risk of death than standard Kt/V. J Am Soc Nephrol 1991; 2: 318.
35. Hakim RM, Lawrence P, Schulman G, Breyer J, Ismail N. Increasing dose of dialysis improves mortality and nutritional parameters in hemodialysis patients. J Am Soc Nephrol 1992; 3: 367.
36. Charra B, Calemard E, Ruffet M, et al. Survival as an index of adequacy of dialysis. Kidney Int 1992; 41: 1286–1291.
37. Kramer P, Broyer M, Brunner FP, et al. Combined report on regular dialysis and transplantation in Europe, XII, 1981. Proc Eur Dial Transplant Assoc 1983; 19: 4–59.
38. Wizemann V, Kramer W. Short-term dialysis – Long-term complications: Ten years experience with short-duration renal replacement therapy. Blood Purif 1987; 5: 193–201.
39. Scribner BH. Editorial: adequate control of blood pressure in patients on chronic hemodialysis. Kidney Int 1992; 41: 1286.
40. Cheigh JS, Milite C, Sullivan JF, Rubin AL, Stenzel KH. Hypertension is not adequately controlled in hemodialysis patients. Am J Kidney Dis 1992; 19: 453–459.
41. Fernández JM, Carbonell ME, Mazzuchi N, Petruccelli D. Simultaneous analysis of morbidity and mortality factors in chronic hemodialysis patients.
42. Held PJ, Levin NW, Bovbjerg RR, Pauly MV, Diamond LH. Mortality and duration of hemodialysis treatment. JAMA 1991; 265: 871–875.
43. Barth RH, Rubin JE, Berlyne GM. Very high blood flow rate is safe and effective in hemodialysis. ASAIO Abstr 1988; 17: 58.
44. Ronco C, Feriani M, La Greca G. Hemodynamic response to high blood flows and ultrafiltration modelling during short dialysis. Kidney Int 1990; 37: 317.

45. Barth RH. Dialysis. In Trigg GL, editor. Encyclopedia of Applied Physics, Vol. 4, VCH, 1992, 533–555.
46. Blagg CR: personal communication.
47. Barth RH. Direct calculation of Kt/V: A simplified approach to monitoring of hemodialysis. Nephron 1988; 50: 190–195.
48. Barth RH. Urea modeling and Kt/V: A critical appraisal. Kidney Int 1993 (in press).
49. Galen M. Reasonably short hemodialysis time can be achieved without high-efficiency dialyzers and without ultrafiltration-controlled delivery systems. Trans ASAIO 1989; 35: 255–257.
50. Lim VS, Flanigan MJ, Fangman J. Effect of hematocrit on solute removal during high efficiency hemodialysis. Kidney Int 1990; 37: 1557–1562.
51. Collins DM, Lambert MB, Middleton JP, et al. Fistula dysfunction: Effect on rapid hemodialysis. Kidney Int 1992; 41: 1292–1296.
52. LeFebvre JM, Spanner E, Heidenheim AP, Lindsay RM. Kt/V: Patients do not get what the physician prescribes. ASAIO Trans 1991; 37: M132–M133.

CHAPTER 15

Functional and vocational rehabilitation of hemodialysis patients

ONYEKACHI IFUDU, HENRY PAUL, JOAN MAYERS,
LINDA COHEN, WILLIAM F. BREZSNYAK, ALLEN HERMAN,
MORRELL M. AVRAM and ELI A. FRIEDMAN

Introduction

End-stage renal disease, is unique in being the only major chronic illness whose cost of care is funded by the government with the criteria solely based on diagnosis [1]. At its inception in 1971 few demographers or policy makers anticipated that the program would grow to its current level in terms of cost [2–4]. In the seventies and eighties, a series of studies on the rehabilitation of hemodialysis patients was done, the results of which showed both suboptimal physical activity and low employment rate [5,6]. Then employment was used as a major index of rehabilitation, primarily because the policy makers who passed the bill were convinced that a great number of hemodialysis patients would be vocationally rehabilitated thereby contributing to the tax base [1]. While several studies have found that the latter objective has not been achieved, other investigators have found improved 'quality of life' especially with the controlled use of erythropoietin in study settings [7,8]. In the current atmosphere of health care reform and fiscal austerity we revisit the issue of functional and vocational rehabilitation of maintenance hemodialysis patients, by a multicenter survey of a large number of patients but this time under real life conditions of erythropoietin use.

Methods and subjects

Subjects

Data was collected from 430 randomly selected maintenance hemodialysis patients, in six Brooklyn ambulatory hemodialysis units (2 hospital-based units; 4 free-standing not-for-profit units) and two ambulatory hemodialysis units in suburban New Jersey (1 hospital-based and 1 free-standing). We

159

E. A. Friedman (ed.), Death on Hemodialysis, 159–167.
© 1994 *Kluwer Academic Publishers.*

Table 1. Modified Karnofsky scale

Activity	Score
Normal function, no disability	96–100
Minor signs and symptoms, full activity	91–95
Usual activities with effort	81–94
Independent, most out of home activities	76–80
Independent, limited to home	70–75
Needs assistance with errands	65–69
Needs assistance with meal preparation	60–64
Needs assistance with bathing/dressing	55–59
Home attendant, not totally disabled	50–54
Disabled, living at home	45–49
Nursing home for chronic care	40–44
Hospitalized, fair condition	35–39
Hospitalized, poor condition	30–34
Hospitalized, progressive fatal process	< 30

interviewed only patients who had been on maintenance hemodialysis for at least 12 months. A cohort of 20 patients were reinterviewed by a different investigator to validate the reproducibility of the scoring system. The survey was conducted by two physicians and two nurses, and to minimize error and ensure high-quality data, they were all intensively instructed before proceeding with data collection. All interviews were performed on site within the various dialysis units.

Information collected from each subject included: Age, gender, race, etiology of ESRD, years on hemodialysis, highest educational level achieved, number of treatments missed in the last two months due to noncompliance, type of health insurance, prior kidney transplants, whom does patient live with, recombinant erythropoietin therapy, and vocational status (employed outside the home; full-time student or full-time homemaker). The most recent predialysis blood chemistry tests including serum creatinine, serum albumin, and hematocrit were reviewed.

Objective parameters

Functional status. We utilized a modified Karnofsky activity scale [9] to assess level of physical activity. Due to the potential pitfalls in the Karnofsky scale [10], we modified it to have fourteen different levels of activity ranging from < 30 (hospitalized, progressive fatal process) to ≥ 96 (Normal function, no disability), narrowing the range at each level to minimize observer variation (Table 1). A score of below seventy indicated that the subject was unable to perform routine living chores without assistance.

Hospitalization. Patient interview was complemented by reviewing medical records to get the number of times patient was hospitalized in the last one year, reason for each hospitalization, and whether each hospital stay was less

Table 2. Demographic profile and laboratory data (n = 430)

Mean age, years (range)	56±14 (21–92)
Gender, Men/Women	215/215
Diabetics	157 (36.5%)
Nodiabetics	273
Number of patients aged 50 years and over	283 (66%)
Mean duration on MD (years) (range)	4.09±3.8 (1–23)
Race	
Black	280 (65%)
White	114 (27%)
Hispanic	27
Asian	9
Level of education	
Below high school	121
High school	237
College	72 (17%)
Serum creatinine (mg/dL)	12.2±3.9
Hematocrit (%)	29±4.5
Serum albumin (g/dL)	3.7±0.4

or more than one week.

Comorbidity index. The presence of significant medical conditions or disability associated with major organ systems was documented. Each medical condition was assigned the number 1, and a numerical comorbidity index generated by totalling the medical conditions present in each patient. The presence of any one of the following was noted: cancer, use of walking aide, congestive heart failure, amputation, angina, blindness, obstructive airway disease, stroke, wheelchair use, arthritis, bone disease, endocrine disease, bowel disease, neuropsychiatric disease and blood disease. We concede that there may be flaws in such an index since the severity of each condition is not taken into consideration. The maximum possible comorbidity index for each subject was 15.

Statistical analysis

Comparison of groups for statistical significance was performend using paired or non-paired Student's *t* test where applicable. Chi-square analysis was used for comparison of within group changes. Unless otherwise indicated, all plus-minus values are mean ± standard deviation.

Results

A total of 430 patients were studied. Mean age of the study group was 56 ± 14 years (range 21–92 yrs) as shown in Table 2. There were 215 men and 215 women and the racial distribution was as follows: 280 (65%) blacks, 114 (27%) whites, 27 (6%) hispanics, and 9 (2%) Asians. Renal diagnoses in the study subjects were: hypertension 162, diabetes mellitus 157, chronic glomerulonephritis 21, adult polycystic kidney disease 15, systemic lupus erythematosus 14, heroin nephropathy 9, obstructive nephropathy 8, drug toxicity 5, congenital kidney disease 4, sickle cell disease 1, and unknown 34. Mean duration of maintenance hemodialysis was 4.09±3.8 years (range 1–23 years). 72 (17%) had a college level education, while 237 (55%) had completed high school, and 121 (28%) had less than a high school education. 42 (10%) of the 430 patients missed a total of 96 dialysis treatments due to noncompliance in the two months prior to the survey (range 1–8 missed dialysis treatments). Medical insurance coverage was provided only by Medicaid for 84, only by Medicare for 65, by both Medicare and Medicaid for 132, private insurance 16, and by Medicare and private insurance for 111, while 22 had all three coverages. Of the 430 patients surveyed only 26 have ever received a kidney transplant. One patient had two prior kidney transplants in the past, while another had three prior kidney transplants. Regarding living arrangements, 417 patients lived at home and 13 resided in a chronic care facility. Of the 417 that live at home, 318 lived with their family or a friend, 63 lived alone and 36 lived with a home attendant. 376 (87%) of 430 patients were on recombinant erythropoietin therapy. Values for predialysis laboratory tests were: serum creatinine 12.2±3.9 mg/dL; serum albumin 3.7±0.4 g/dL; and hematocrit 29±4.5 percent.

Vocational status

Only 3 of the subjects studied were full-time students. 70 (16%) patients were full-time homemakers, and 43 (10%) patients were employed outside the home. The college educated patients were more likely to be employed outside the home – possibly in part to the likelihood of their being more likely to be in sedentary, less-physically tasking jobs. While 21 (29%) of 72 college-educated subjects were employed outside the home, only 16 (7%) of 237 with high school education, and 6 (5%) of 121 subjects with less than high school education were employed outside the home (p = 0.0001). Furthermore of 193 patients aged < 65 years, who were deemed physically capable (i.e. modified Karnofsky score ≥ 76 = independent, participating in most out of home activities) of working, only 26 (13%) were employed outside the home. The reason often proffered by most of the latter group, was the fear of losing all or part of their health insurance benefits or their disability rating if they get a job.

Functional status

154 (36%) of 430 patients had scored < 70 on the modified Karnofsky scale – meaning that they were unable to perform routine living chores without assistance (Table 3). Reliance on a wheelchair to get around for all or part of the day was reported by 73 (17%) of the study group. As a group, diabetic

Table 3. Functional and vocational status

	Number of patients
Unable to perform routine living chores without assistance (i.e. modified Karnofsky score < 70)	154 (36%)
Use of wheelchair	73 (17%)
Living with home attendant	36 (8.4%)
Employed outside the home	43 (10%)
Full-time homemaker	70 (16%)
Full-time student	3

Table 4. Diabetic subjects vs nondiabetic subjects

	Diabetics (n = 157)	Nondiabetics (n = 273)	P
Mean age (years)	61.3±10.4	54±16	0.001
Number of patients unable to perform routine living chores without assistance	86 (55%)	68 (25%)	0.0001
Number of pts using a wheelchair	45 (29%)	28 (10%)	0.001
Mean comorbidity index	2.4±1.7	1.4±1.4	0.0001
Number of pts hospitalized at least once in the past 1 year	103 (66%)	157 (58%)	0.46
Total number of hospitalizations	212	296	0.006
Mean number of hospitalizations	1.34±1.4	1.1±1.3	0.7
Percent of hospital admissions with length of stay > 1 week	69%	59%	0.3

patients had a worse outcome than their nondiabetic counterparts (Table 4). 86 (55%) of 157 diabetic patients were unable to perform routine living chores without assistance as against 68 (25%) of 273 nondiabetic patients (p = 0.0001). Also 45 (29%) of 157 diabetic patients were wheelchair bound compared to 28 (10%) of nondiabetic patients who were dependent on a wheelchair to get around (p = 0.001). However, when stratified into age groups as shown in Table 5 there is a paucity of diabetic patients below age 50 years, and the diabetic patients who were significantly more functionally impaired than their nondiabetic counterparts, were those in the 50–59 age group.

Hospitalization

260 (60%) of the 430 patients surveyed accounted for a total of 508 hospitalizations for various ailments in the past 1 year. Length of stay was more than one week for 322 (63%) of the hospital admissions. Though the diabetic subjects were hospitalized more often (1.34±1.4) than the nondiabetic subjects (1.1±1.3) (p = 0.7), and were more likely to spend more time when

Table 5. Number of patients in each age group who were unable to perform routine living chores without assistance (i.e. Modified Karnofsky scores < 70)

	Diabetics (n = 157)	Nondiabetics (n = 273)	P
20–29 n=0 D & 14 ND)	–	4	–
30–39 n=5 D & 50 ND)	2	4	0.27
40–49 n=12 D & 66 ND)	1	4	0.7
50–59 n=47 D & 41 ND)	19	4	0.02
60+ n=93 D & 102 ND)	64	52	0.25

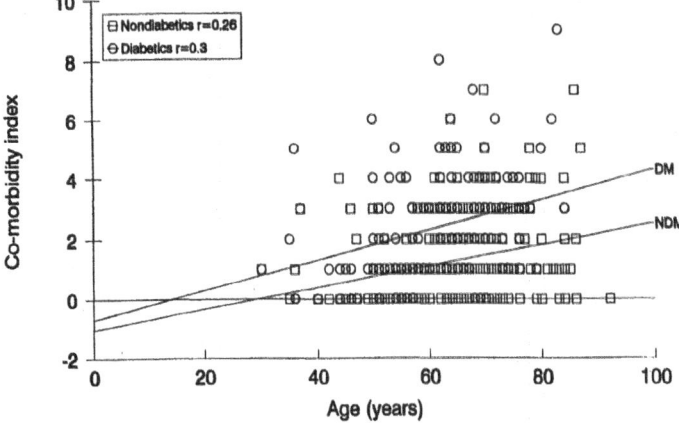

Fig. 1.   Age and comorbidity index.

admitted (69% of all hospital admissions > 1 week) than the nondiabetic subjects (59% of all admissions > 1 week) (p = 0.3), these differences were not statistically significant (Table 4).

Comorbidity index

The mean comorbidity index for the entire study group was 1.7 ± 1.6. Comorbid medical conditions were more prevalent in diabetic subjects with a mean comorbidity index of 2.4 ± 1.7 as against a comorbidity index of 1.4 ± 1.4 in the nondiabetic subjects (p = 0.0001) (Table 4). As shown in Fig. 1, the comorbidity index increased with advancing age, but the correlation is not very strong.

Impact of race

A summary of comparisons between white and black diabetic subjects is shown in Table 6. Regarding functional status, more of the white diabetic

Table 6. Impact of race

	Black diabetics (n = 101)	White diabetics (n = 39)	*P*
Mean age (years)	59.8±10	67.3±8.4	0.001
Number of patients unable to perform routine living chores without assistance	44 (44%)	30 (70%)	0.08
Number of hospitalizations	1.34±1.4	1.33±1.3	0.9
Comorbidity index	2.4±1.7	2.5±1.8	0.7

subjects, 30 (70%) of 39 required assistance to perform routine living chores than the black diabetic subjects 44 (44%) of 101, but this difference was not statistically significant (p = 0.08). There was a significant difference in the mean age of the two groups (black diabetic subjects 59.8±10 years; white diabetic subjects 67.3±8.4 years, (p = 0.001). Both groups had equivalent number of hospitalizations and similar comorbidity indices.

Discussion

Our results show that only 10 percent of the patients surveyed were employed outside the home while 16 percent were full time home makers. This represents a sharp decline from studies in the early eighties that found 25% of ESRD patients to be employed [5]. Viewed from a different perspective, of the 193 patients aged < 65 who were deemed functionally able (modified Karnofsky score ≥ 76) only 26 (13%) were employed outside the home. One recurring theme among this group was anxiety over forfeiture of medical benefits and disability rating should they become employed. The effect of the prevailing economic downturn on the employment data is unclear.

Regarding functional status, 36% of the patients required assistance with routine daily chores and 8.4% were so constrained that they needed a home attendant. Diabetics patients had a worse outcome than did nondiabetic patients in most of the objective indicators utilized, most notably, functional status as measured by the modified Karnofsky scale.

The reasons for the continued poor functional status and low rates of employment are uncertain. In the two decades since the initiation of the Medicare ESRD program, some profound changes have occurred in the field of Nephrology and its client population. The influence of these changes on our findings is unclear, because examined individually, the impact of some of these changes can be easily discerned, but the outcome of all the factors acting in concert is not easily predictable. Clearly, on the upside is the emergence and the wide use of recombinant human erythropoietin, improvement in dialyzer and dialysate technology, and the influence of ESRD patient advocacy groups [2,11]. There have also been improvements in drug therapy of some features of uremia like renal osteodystrophy with parenteral calcitriol, resulting from research that debunked old practices by revealing precise pathogenesis [12]. Added to these, is that nephrologists have acquired a lot of expertise in the care of their patients.

On the downside, however, is that new starts on maintenance hemodialysis are now older than before, with the mean age in 1991 being 56.6 years [2]. In addition, the new starts now tend to be sicker since the prevalence of comorbid medical conditions is higher in the older patients than in their younger counterparts [2,13]. Furthermore, there are now more diabetic patients than ever before receiving renal replacement therapy [2], and most distressing is the new craze of shortening dialysis time disguised by its practitioners as pro-efficiency, but viewed by others as an exercise driven by less than pristine motives.

The impact of the proposed health care reform on the ESRD program is unclear, but our findings are instructive and may be valuable in devising guidelines for governmental funding of life-prolonging therapy in the chronically ill. Patients who have chronic illness are under major physical and psychological burdens, and a realistic approach regarding the goals of therapy and potential for both functional and vocational rehabilitation should be taken. Physicians, in their desire to be advocates for their patients, need not be driven to give assurances to third party payers as to future rehabilitation status of the patient, before medical coverage could be provided. This is pertinent since patients entering the ESRD program are now older and it is projected that by the year 2000 the mean age of the new dialysis patient will be 60 years [2]. Secondly, there is a need to incorporate into health care reform, measures to ensure that ESRD patients or patients with other chronic illnesses who are physically fit and decide to work, do no lose part or all of their medical benefits.

In the meantime efforts need to be devoted towards maximizing the use of available resources to achieve excellent functional rehabilitation in ESRD patients, because life is much more than survival.

References

1. Gutman RA. High-cost life prolongation: the national kidney dialysis and transplantation study. Ann Intern Med 1988; 108: 898–899.
2. US Renal Data System. USRDS 1990 Annual Report. Bethesda, MD: National Institutes of Health, National Institute of Diabetes and Digestive and Kidney Diseases; 1990.
3. Friedman EA, Delano BG, Butt KMH. Pragmatic realities in uremia therapy. N Engl J Med 1978; 298: 368–371.
4. Iglehart JK. The American health care system – The end-stage renal disease program. N Engl J Med 1993; 328: 366–371.
5. Gutman RA, Stead WW, Robinson RR. Physical activity and employment status of patients on maintenance hemodialysis. N Engl J Med 1981; 304: 309–313.
6. Evans RW, Manninen DL, Garrison LP, Hart G, Blagg BR, Gutman RA, Hull AR, Lowrie EG. The quality of life of patients with end-stage renal disease. N Engl J Med 1985; 312: 553–559.
7. Carlson DM, Johnson WJ, Kjellstrand CM. Functional status of patients with end-stage renal disease. Mayo Clin Proc 1987; 62: 338–344.

8. Evans RW, Rader B, Manninen DL and the Cooperative Multicenter EPO Clinical Trial Group. JAMA 1990; 263: 825–830.
9. Karnofsky DA, Burchenal JH. The clinical evaluation of chemotherapeutic agents in cancer. In: Macleod CM, editor. Evaluation of chemotherapeutic agents. New York: Columbia University Press, 1949: 191–205.
10. Hutchinson TA, Boyd NF, Feinstein AR. Scientific problems in clinical scales, as demonstrated in the Karnofsky index of performance status. J. Chronic Dis. 1979; 32: 661–666.
11. Eschbach JW, Egrie JC, Downing MR, Browne JK, Adamson JW. Correction of anemia of end-stage renal disease with recombinant human erythropoietin. N Eng J Med 1987; 316: 73–78.
12. Delmez JA, Slatopolsky E. Recent advances in the pathogenesis and therapy of uremic secondary hyperparathyroidism. J Clin Endocrinol Metab 1991; 72: 735–739.
13. Shapiro FL, Umen AJ. Risk factors in hemodialysis patient survival. Am Assoc Artif Intern Organs J 1983; 6: 176–184.

CHAPTER 16

Correlates of long-term survival on hemodialysis

MORRELL M. AVRAM, PHILIP GOLDWASSER,
DANUTA DERKATZ and SARA-ANN GUSIK

Introduction

The high mortality of hemodialysis (HD) patients in the United States has prompted an examination of causes and markers of mortality risk [1–15]. The National Cooperative Dialysis study demonstrated reduced morbidity in patients randomized to receive high urea clearances (i.e. treatments designed to maintain low serum urea nitrogen [BUN] levels) in the context of adequate protein intake [6]. Yet, the opposite was found in later cross-sectional studies of HD patients. Increased survival was found to be associated with high BUN and creatinine values [6–12]. Lowrie and Lew reported that one-year mortality risk was increased independently by low serum albumin, creatinine and cholesterol as well as age and male gender [11]. They also noted that the association of diabetes with mortality risk was diminished by statistical adjustment for the serum nutritional profile, particularly the concentrations of creatinine and albumin [11,12]. We found that single measurements of albumin and creatinine are independent predictors of survival for up to two years in both recently-diagnosed and longstanding HD patients even when adequately dialyzed [13]. Whether certain markers are correlated more strongly with short term risk vs long term risk remains to be studied.

We now report an analysis of the survival experience of 221 HD patients monitored for up to 58 months. The correlates of early mortality risk, late mortality, and long term survival were determined by multinomial logistic regression. To examine the nutritional markers of apparently stable patients, four-year trends of nutritional markers (weight, serum albumin and creatinine) were examined in long term survivors.

169

E. A. Friedman (ed.), Death on Hemodialysis, 169–176.
© 1994 Kluwer Academic Publishers. Printed in the Netherlands.

Methods

Patient enrollment and follow-up

Two hundred twenty-one HD outpatients were enrolled in annual cohorts between 1987 and 1991 (June 1987 n = 82, April 1988 n = 35, April 1989 n = 50, February 1990 n = 19, February 1991 n = 35). The patients were monitored until April 1, 1992 (mean 26 months, median 23 months, maximum 58 months). Patients previously on CAPD were not enrolled. Follow-up was censored on transplantation, switch to CAPD, or transfer to another center.

Baseline and follow-up data

At enrollment, clinical, demographic and biochemical data were recorded for new cases. At the same time, follow-up measurements of biochemical data were recorded for previously enrolled patients. This resulted in serial data for many subjects. Blood drawn from the arteriovenous access before beginning the treatment session was tested for BUN, creatinine, albumin and cholesterol using the SMAC autoanalyzer (Technicon, Tarrytown, NY).

Mean age at enrollment was 59 ± 16 [SD] years, and mean prior months on HD was 37 ± 42. At enrollment, diabetic patients had been on dialysis for fewer months than non-diabetic patients (29 ± 33 vs 42 ± 47, p < 0.04). Fifty-five percent (55%) of the patients were female; thirty-nine percent (39%) had diabetes. The racial composition was fifty-four percent (54%) black, thirty percent (30%) white, sixteen percent (16%) Hispanic. The causes of ESRD were: hypertension (36%), diabetes (34%), primary glomerular disease (8%), polycystic disease (7%), urologic (3%), lupus or vasculitis (3%), miscellaneous (6%), and unknown (3%).

Study design and data analysis

For the survival study, the patients were divided into three groups by outcome: group I died ≤ 12 months after enrollment (n = 42); Group II died 13–58 months after enrollment (n = 59); group III survived > 24 months before follow-up was censored (n = 77). Cases with ≤ 24 months of follow-up prior to censorship were excluded from this analysis (n = 43). Using group III as reference group, a model was constructed by multinomial logistic regression that predicts the likelihood of group I (vs III) and group II (vs III). Prior months on dialysis was included in the model to adjust for length-selection bias.

For the trend study, serial measurements of weight, albumin and creatinine were examined over four years in subjects who (i) enrolled in 1987; (ii) had serial measurements recorded every year through 1991; (iii) underwent no major amputation surgery during 1987–1991; and (iv) survived > 11 months after the final sampling. Twenty-eight patients (seven with diabetes) satisfied

Table 1. Baseline characteristics by outcome

	Early death (41)	Late death (59)	Survivors (77)	P
Age	66 ± 12	63 ± 14	54 ± 15	$< 10^{-4}$
Months on dialysis	37 ± 44	43 ± 45	41 ± 46	0.57
Weight (lb.)	140 ± 33	143 ± 39	145 ± 28	0.21
Race				
White (%)	39%	27%	21%	
Black (%)	51%	58%	56%	
Hispanic (%)	10%	15%	23%	
Male (%)	32%	39%	55%	0.04
Diabetes (%)	51%	40%	29%	0.05
Albumin (gm/dl)	3.50 ± 0.50	3.81 ± 0.43	4.00 ± 0.33	$< 10^{-4}$
Creatinine (mg/dl)	10.75 ± 4.65	13.24 ± 5.24	15.00 ± 4.57	$< 10^{-4}$
BUN (mg/dl)	77.8 ± 24.5	86.5 ± 21.8	89.0 ± 24.9	0.052
Cholesterol (mg/dl)	171.4 ± 52.8	169.2 ± 42.3	189.4 ± 50.1	0.033

these criteria. Trends were examined for this entire group and for subgroups by diabetic status. Comparisons were made using the paired t-test.

For comparisons of means and proportions between groups, ANOVA, the Kruskal-Wallis test, and the Chi-square test were used as appropriate.

Computations were performed using SPSS 5.0.2 for Windows and SYSTAT statistical software.

Results

Long term survival vs early and late death

The clinical and biochemical characteristics of the patients stratified by outcome status are shown in Table 1. Variables associated with increased mortality risk were age, female gender, diabetes and lower concentrations of serum albumin, creatinine, cholesterol and BUN.

Owing to potential confounding among factors identified in univariate analysis, the independent predictors of outcome were determined with multinomial logistic regression. The model estimates the likelihood of death one year or less after enrollment (n = 41), or 13–58 months after enrollment (n = 59) relative to a reference group of survivors who received more than two years of follow-up. Variables with significant independent predictive value included age, diabetes and serum albumin and cholesterol (Tables 2 and 3).

Adjusting for the other variables, age at enrollment increased the odds of death by 5–6% per year. Both serum albumin and cholesterol correlated directly with prognosis, although serum albumin was more strongly correlated with early risk and serum cholesterol with late risk. For each 1 gm/dl increase in baseline serum albumin, the relative odds of early death fell by 93% ($p<10^{-3}$) and that of late death by 60% (p <0.10). For each 1 mg/dl increase

Table 2. Predictors of early death ($\leq$ 12 months) vs survival for > 2 years (Multinomial logistic regression)

Predictor	Regression coefficient ($\pm$ SE)	ratio	P
Age (per year)	0.056 ± 0.019	1.06	0.003
Months of HD			
13–60 (vs $\leq$ 12)	0.27 ± 0.55	1.31	0.014
> 60 (vs $\leq$ 12)	0.95 ± 0.63	2.59	0.133
Albumin (per gm/dl)	–2.60 ± 0.61	0.073	<0.001
Cholesterol (per mg/dl)	–0.009 ± 0.005	0.99	.071
Diabetes	0.97 ± 0.47	2.64	0.04

Table 3. Predictors of late death (1–5 years) vs survival for > 2 years (Multinomial logistic regression)

Predictors	Regression coefficient ($\pm$ SE)	ratio	P
Age (per year)	0.052 ± 0.015	1.05	0.001
Months of HD			
13–60 (vs $\leq$ 12)	0.66 ± 0.46	1.94	0.146
> 60 (vs $\leq$ 12)	0.64 ± 0.55	1.89	0.243
Albumin (per gm/dl)	–0.91 ± 0.54	0.40	0.093
Cholesterol (per mg/dl)	–0.011 ± 0.004	0.99	0.009
Diabetes	0.45 ± 0.41	1.57	0.265

in baseline serum cholesterol, there was a 1% reduction in the relative risk of early death (p x 0.07) and of late death (p x 0.009).

Diabetes was associated with a two-to-three-fold increase in early death risk (p x 0.04), and a less significant increase in late risk (odds ratio 1.57 p x 0.27). In the model for early risk (Table 2), creatinine was a significant correlate of survival (p <0.05) if diabetes was not used in the model. If diabetes and creatinine were used in the model, neither was significant (p <0.15). Fewer months on dialysis was associated with better prognosis although the effect was not statistically significant.

Table 4. Biochemical and weight trends over 4 years in 28 stable patients

Year	Albumin (gm/dl)	Creatinine (gm/dl)	Weight (lbs)
1987	4.03 ± 0.36	16.98 ± 3.83	143 ± 23
1988	4.03 ± 0.37	16.02 ± 3.49	145 ± 23
1989	3.94 ± 0.36	15.41 ± 2.69	145 ± 22
1990	3.88 ± 0.33	14.95 ± 3.03	145 ± 22
1991	3.82 ± 0.23*	14.12 ± 2.57*	144 ± 21

* 1987 vs 1991 p $\leq$ 0.001 by paired t-test

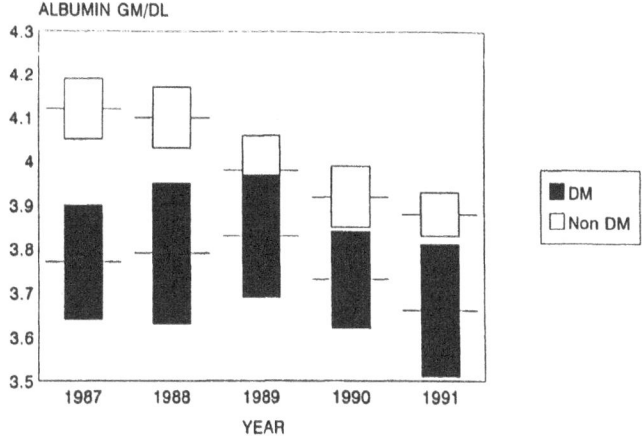

Fig. 1. Albumin concentration trend in 21 nondiabetic and 7 diabetic patients.

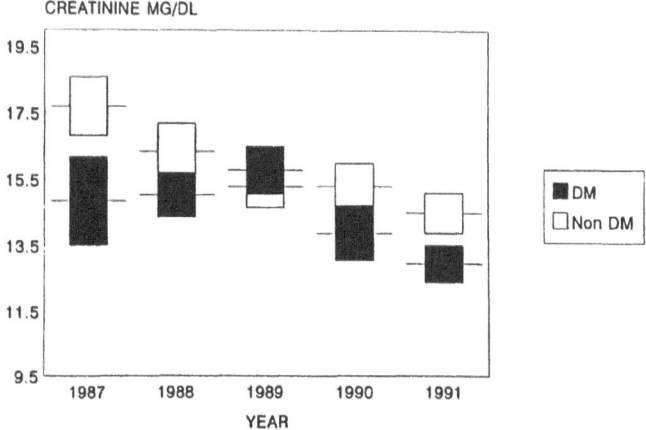

Fig. 2. Creatinine concentration trend in 21 nondiabetic and 7 diabetic patients.

Trends

Estimated dry weight did not change over four years (Table 4). Both albumin ($p < 0.001$) and creatinine (p x 0.001) fell significantly over four years (1987 vs 1991) (Table 4). The trends were similar in nondiabetic (n x 21) and diabetic subjects (n x 7) (Figs. 1–3). Although the values of albumin and creatinine fell over time for both diabetic and non-diabetic subgroups, the comparison of 1987 to 1991 values were not significant for the diabetic subgroup, in part due to its smaller size.

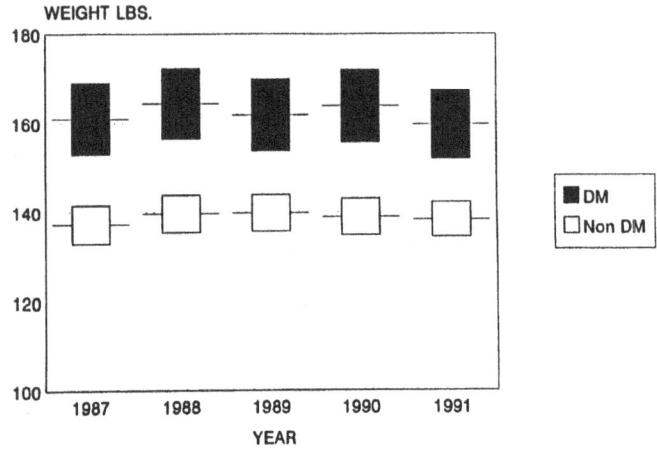

Fig. 3.   Weight trend in 21 nondiabetic and 7 diabetic patients.

Discussion

Malnutrition is prevalent in ESRD patients [14,15,16,17]. Certain subgroups such as patients with diabetes, are particularly prone to nutritional depletion. The serum markers of visceral protein status include albumin and cholesterol (reflecting lipoproteins) [18]. Serum creatinine reflects both somatic protein status and dialysis dose, and BUN reflects both recent protein intake as well as dialysis dose. Studies have found strong direct correlations between the concentrations of these markers and the prognosis of HD and CAPD patients over one-two years [7–13]. The present report examined the relationship of baseline concentrations of albumin, creatinine, cholesterol and BUN to long-term survival (2–5 years) vs early (≤ 1 year) or late (2–5 years) mortality. In addition, the nutritional markers of 'stable' HD patients was examined over a four-year period.

The survival study extends our previous report of four year survival by exploring the relationship of these markers to different survival periods [15]. The findings were consistent with the previous report in that albumin and cholesterol were important predictors of survival. Albumin was particularly important ($p < 0.001$) in identifying patients at early risk, and was less significant ($p < 0.10$) in differentiating late deaths from survival. Cholesterol was more significant in differentiating late risk. Patients with diabetes were at more than two-fold increased risk ($p \times 0.04$) for death in the first year after study enrollment, but only at 50% increased risk of late death. Creatinine concentration could replace diabetes in the model, although it was somewhat less significant. This suggests that creatinine reflects an aspect of mortality risk that is characteristic of diabetes, e.g. reduced somatic protein.

The influence of predictors on the risk of late death (Table 3) were generally consistent with their effect on early death (Table 1), although in the case of albumin and diabetes, less significant. Whether this reflects the length-selection bias intrinsic to the study, or true biologic differences in the correlates of early and late mortality risk cannot be stated.

Given the prognostic importance of protein status, we examined whether apparently stable HD patients have stable protein status. The results show a disturbing decline in visceral and somatic protein status (reflected in serum albumin and creatinine, respectively). The observed trends are compatible with the downward trend in apoprotein B concentrations we reported in HD and PD patients [19]. These changes in protein status were masked by a lack of change in estimated dry weight suggesting a possible alteration in body composition over time. The trends are steeper than would be expected from aging alone and therefore, may be the result of the catabolic tendency of CRF patients or inadequacy of renal replacement therapy [20,21].

To summarize, age, diabetes, and reduced concentrations of albumin and cholesterol are important predictors of mortality risk in HD. The findings are consistent with the hypothesis that protein-energy malnutrition is the main cause of mortality in ESRD. Our findings also suggest that even apparently stable patients are at nutritional risk. Further research should be directed to improving the nutritional intake and decreasing the catabolism of dialysis patients.

Summary

The correlates of long term survival on dialysis were examined in 221 patients monitored for up to five years. The variables examined included demographics, cause of ESRD and serum urea, creatinine, albumin and cholesterol. Using multinomial logistic regression, a model was derived that discriminated long term survivors (with more than two years of follow up compared with early [≤ 1 year] and late [1–5 year] deaths). Age, albumin, and diabetes were most strongly correlated with late risk.

In a second study, we examined the four year trends (1987–1991) of weight and serum albumin and cholesterol in 28 patients who enrolled in 1987 and survived until 1992. Despite their clinical stability, serum albumin and creatinine, but not weight, trended downwards.

In conclusion, age, diabetes and albumin and cholesterol are important prognostic factors over one to five years. Even apparently stable patients may be at nutritional risk.

References

1. End-Stage Renal Disease Program Facility Survey Tables 1982 through 1988. Baltimore MD. ESRD Information Analysis Branch, Division of Information Analysis, Health Care Financing Administration: 1989.

2. Hull AR, Parker TF III Proceedings from the Morbidity, Mortality and Prescriptions of Dialysis Symposium, Dallas TX, September 15 to 17, 1989, Am J Kidney Dis 1990: 15: 375–383.

3. United States Renal Data System, USRDS 1989 Annual Report. Bethesda, MD, National Institutes of Health, National Institute of Diabetes and Digestive and Kidney Diseases: August, 1989.

4. Held PJ, Brunner F, Odaka M, Garcia JR, Port FK, Gaylin DS. Five-year survival for end-stage renal disease patients in the United States, Europe, and Japan, 1982 to 1987. Am J Kidney Dis 1990; 15: 451–457.

5. Gotch FA, Vehlinger DE. Mortality rate in US dialysis patients. Dial Transplant 1991; 20: 255–257.

6. Laird NM, Berkey CS, Lowrie EG. Modeling success or failure of dialysis therapy. The National Cooperative Dialysis Study. Kidney Int 1983; 23 (Suppl 13): S101–S106.

7. Acchiardo SR, Moore LW, Latour PA. Malnutrition as the main factor in morbidity and mortality of dialysis patients. Kidney Int 1983; 24 (Suppl 16): S199–S203.

8. Avram MM, Slater PA, Gan A, et al. Predialysis BUN and creatinine do not predict adequate dialysis, clinical rehabilitation, or longevity. Kidney Int 1985; 28: S100–S104.

9. Shapiro JI, Argy WB, Rakowski TA, Chester A, Siemsen AS, Schreiner GA: The unsuitability of BUN as a criterion for prescription dialysis. Trans Am Soc Artif Organs 1983; 29: 129–132.

10. Cano N, Fernandez JP, Lacombe P, et al.. Statistical selection of nutritional parameters in hemodialyzed patients. Kidney Int 1987; 32: (Suppl 22): S178–S180.

11. Lowrie EG, Lew NL. Death risk in hemodialysis patients: The predictive value of commonly measured variables and an evaluation of the death rate differences between facilities. Am J Kidney Dis 1990; 15: 458–482.

12. Lowrie EG, Lew NL, Huang WH. Race and diabetes as death risk predictors in hemodialysis patients. Kidney Int 1992; 42 (S 38): S22–S31.

13. Goldwasser P, Mittman N, Antignani A, Burrell D, Michel M, Collier J, Avram MM. Predictors of mortality in hemodialysis patients. J Am Soc Neph 1993; 3(9): 1613–1622.

14. Steinman TI and Mitch WE. Nutrition in dialysis patients. In: Maher JF, editor. Replacement of renal function by dialysis. Dordrecht, Holland: Kluwer Academic Publ, 1989: 1088–1106.

15. Wolfsori M, Strong CJ, Minturn D, et al. Nutritional status and lymphocyte function in maintenance hemodialysis patients. Am J Clin Nutr 1984; 39: 547–555.

16. Young GA, Swanepoel CR, Craft MR, et al. Anthropometry and plasma valine, amino acids and proteins in the nutritional assessment of hemodialysis patients. Kidney Int 1982; 21: 492–499.

17. Schoenfeld PY, Henry RR, Laird NM, et al. Assessment of nutritional status of the National Cooperative Dialysis Study population. Kidney Int 1983; 23 (Suppl 13): S80–S88.

18. Torun B, Viteri FE. Protein-energy malnutrition. In: Shils ME, Young VR, editors. Modern Nutrition in Health and Disease. 7th Ed. Philadelphia, Lea Febiger, 1988: 746–773.

19. Avram MM, Goldwasser P, Burrell DE, Antignani A, Fein PA, Mittman N. The uremic dyslipidemia: A cross-sectional and longitudinal study. Am J Kidney Dis 1992; Vol XX No 4 (October): 324–335.

20. Salive ME, Cornoni-Huntley J, Phillips CL et al: Serum albumin in older persons: relationship with age and health status. J Clin Epid 1992; 45: 213–222.

21. Kopple JD: Causes of catabolism and wasting in acute or chronic renal failure. In: Robinson R, editor, Nephrology. New York, Springer-Verlag, 1984: 1498–1514.

CHAPTER 17

Resuscitate home hemodialysis

BARBARA G. DELANO

Introduction

Hemodialysis was first performed in the home in 1964 and 1965 [1,2]. Advantages of cost [3], convenience and enhanced survival [4] were rapidly associated with home hemodialysis. This treatment grew to encompass 42% of all patients in the United States treated for end stage renal disease [5]. In areas of strong advocacy by Nephrologists such as Seattle, the percentage of patients on this therapy was even higher. Shortly after Medicare assumed funding for most treatments of dialysis patients, home hemodialysis began a decline which has continued to the present. Currently less than 2% of the US population is treated in this way [6].

In this paper we will examine what has happened to home hemodialysis, consider why it should be resuscitated and discuss some ideas of how to do this.

Home hemodialysis in the US and elsewhere

The percentage of dialysis patients being treated by hemodialysis at home varies widely from country to country. Data from the 1993 USRDS annual report (Fig. 1) shows a disparity of 0.2% of patients being treated at home in Japan to a high of 21.3% in Australia [6]. With such a disparity in the incidence of this therapy many factors are probably at work. Nissenson and coworkers [7] have recently discussed non-medical factors that impact on uremia treatment modality selection. These are many and include things like cultural factors as in Hong Kong where Chinese patients are more averse to needle punctures than caucasians, as well as small homes in Japan where space considerations would make home hemodialysis impossible. Societal factors such as a significant number of Aborigines in Australia/New Zealand make home hemodialysis difficult. In Canada many patients live far from treatment centers and therefore there is an increase in the incidence of home therapies. Available resources and physician bias also have to be dealt with. If there are many outpatient units available, the tendency for administrators

E. A. Friedman (ed.), Death on Hemodialysis, 177–182.
© 1994 *Kluwer Academic Publishers.*

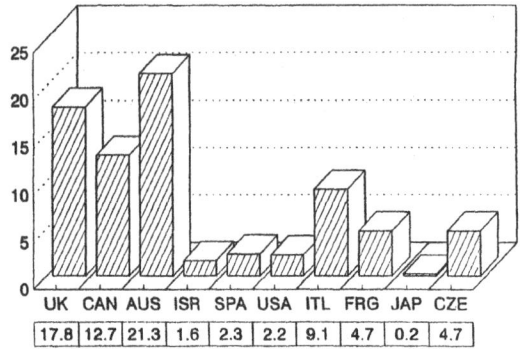

Fig. 1.   The percentage of dialysis patients being treated by home hemodialysis in several countries in 1989. From the USRDS Annual Report 1993.

and owners of those units will be to keep them filled. Those authors also stress the role of financial/reimbursement issues. In countries where there is little or no physician reimbursement for home therapies, the percentage of home dialysis is low. If physicians own dialysis centers it is in their financial interest to refer patients to those units.

Mattern, *et al.* [8] surveyed Nephrologists in 3 different regions, North Carolina, Southern California and Australia/New Zealand to determine their preferences of end stage renal disease therapy. They then determined how patients were assigned to therapy. There was a striking disparity between preferences and practice. Reasons for this are not always apparent, but for example, North Carolina which has 26% of its patients on a home therapy compared to 8% for Southern California has a higher percentage of Academic affiliated Nephrologists (41% vrs 19%).

Even within the United States there is wide variability in the number of patients on home hemodialysis by regional network, varying from 1.8% to 34.1% [9]. The relatively high percentage of home patients in the Washington State area is possible because of a committed staff, expertise, good support services as well as the availability of paid helpers when necessary [10].

If one examines the 5 year cumulative growth rate for the United States from 1984 to 1989 (Fig. 2) [11], home hemodialysis is the only treatment that has declined (8% over 5 years). The most rapid growth has been in peritoneal dialysis, both Chronic Ambulatory Peritoneal Dialysis (CAPD) and Automated Peritoneal Dialysis (APD). These therapies now account for 19% of all dialysis patients in the United States [6]. CAPD is appealing as a home therapy. It is a treatment that can be performed without a helper.

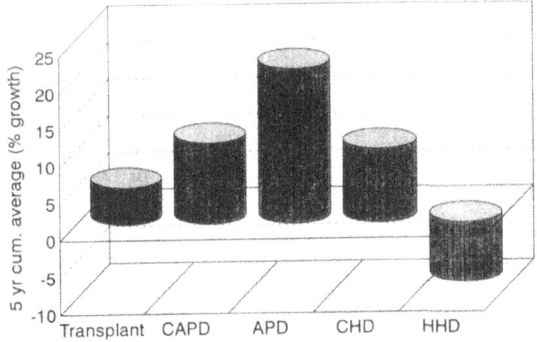

Fig. 2. Five year cumulative average modality growth (%), United States 1984–89. From Inoue R. Cont. Dialysis and Nephrology 1992 [11].

Training time is rapid and most patients can began dialysis in the home after 2 weeks. There is no home modification needed. Medically it may be more suitable for a large segment of the current dialysis population which is increasingly becoming older and sicker [12].

Why resuscitate home hemodialysis?

By almost every measure used, home hemodialysis comes out best of all dialysis therapies. Although there is certainly a selection bias, home hemodialysis offers the best opportunity for long term survival. Rubin, Hsu and Bower [13] had a median survival of 150 home hemodialysis patients of 4030 days. The median survival of patients on limited care dialysis in their facility was 3600 days and 230 CAPD patients had a median survival of 1050 days. Indeed they had a 40% fifteen year home hemodialysis technique survival. Similarly, Mailloux *et al.* [14] analyzing predictors of survival in 532 patients found excellent survival in their home hemodialysis patients (5 and 10 year survival of 90%). They further used the Cox Proportional Hazards Regression Model for data analysis and even correcting for patients age and disease category, survival of patients on home hemodialysis was best. Indeed 19% of the 201 patients we trained for treatment at home remained on this therapy for at least 10 years [15]. Eleven patients were on home hemodialysis for more than 20 years Seven are still receiving dialysis in the home. One received a kidney transplant after 20 years and 3 died, one of aluminum intoxication, one from a myocardial infarction and one from sepsis. These patients are detailed in Table 1.

Table 1. Twenty year survivors on home hemodialysis (HHD)

Pt	Age	Sex/Race	Disease	yrs on HHD	Status
1	57	F/H	IN	28	HHD
2	40	M/W	CONG	24	HHD
3	63	M/B	?	24	HHD
4	47	F/W	CONG	20	HHD
5	47	M/H	HIN	20	HHD
6	63	M/W	HIN	20	HHD
7	42	M/W	?	20	HHD
8	47	M/W	HIN	20	TX
9	60	F/W	IN	22	DIED(SEP)
10	58	F/W	IN	20	DIED(MI)
11	56	F/W	CGN	21	DIED(AL)

HIN = Hereditary Nephritis; AL = Alum. intoxication;
CGN = Chronic Glomerulonephritis; MI = Myocardial Infarction;
IN = Interstial Nephritis; SEP = Sepsis;
CONG = Congenital Disease; TX = Transplant.

Much emphasis has been placed on rehabilitation in dialysis patients. Factors affecting return to work are many and include loss of disability benefits, employer bias and time commitments. Most hemodialysis patients spend at least 10–12 hours per week on the machine. If one includes travel time to and from a unit as well as a treatment scheduled during the day, it is easy to see why routine employment would be difficult. Obviously home hemodialysis patients have an advantage in being able to schedule treatments at their convenience and in saving travel time. While the number of dialysis patients working is low, those patients receiving hemodialysis at home have the highest percentage working (36.2%) or able to work (59.2%) [16]. When all dialysis modalities including in center and peritoneal dialysis are examined, home hemodialysis patients score highest on indexes of well being, happiness, an index of psychological affect, a normal Karnofsky score and perceived health status [17]. This was confirmed in an additional study by Bremer *et al.* [18]. However Rubin, Case and Bower [19] found very similar (and relatively high levels) of rehabilitation when they compared a group of 67 CAPD patients with a group of 76 home hemodialysis patients. If they excluded elderly and debilitated people, full rehabilitation was seen of 57% of the peritoneal group and 65% of the home hemo patients. At this time however, the long term efficacy of CAPD as a therapy is unknown. Only a small number of patients have been on this for more than 5 years. Drop out rates because of repeated episodes of peritonitis or catheter problems, while improving, remain high.

The issue of cost of providing treatment for end stage renal disease is widely discussed. The total cost of the program was $6.6 billion in 1991 [20]. Home treatment, be it peritoneal dialysis or hemo is less expensive than

than in center treatment. A cost effective analysis of varying treatments in New Zealand found an average annual cost of home hemo to be $25,345 compared to $33,125 per in center patient [21]. Data from the National Renal Administrator Association report that the cost of home hemodialysis is approximately $40 less per treatment than outpatient dialysis [22].

How can we resusciate HHD?

Firstly, we have to bring the benefits of home hemodialysis to the attention not only of patients, but of dialysis professionals. Since the number of people on this therapy is so small, many nephrologists may not be familiar with it. One way of doing this is to make a rotation through home training programs a requirement for a renal fellowship. Such a mandate for a rotation through transplantation now exists. Next we have to dispel some of the myths that have become associated with home hemodialysis. Myths that it is not as safe as in center treatment or that no back up is available [23]. Liability issues about responsibility for a helper need to be addressed. Patient groups should take up the banner and increase the awareness of this therapy among other patients, particularly those new to uremia therapy. Next, some new innovative methods must be sought. A major reason for not training some inner city residents in particular is the lack of a suitable partner who can be present throughout every dialysis session. The development of a truly safe machine would obviate the need for a partner, and permit many single people to do their treatments at home.

In summary, there is a serious need to resuscitate home hemodialysis as it offers the best opportunity for a dialysis patient to live a long and productive life. In this age of moving health care into the home it seems ideal. At this time many of the Nephrologists who do advocate home therapy are concentrating on CAPD, but as stated above, the ability of this therapy to be a long term treatment for an end stage renal failure patient remains to be demonstrated.

Summary

Despite having excellent patient and technique survival, home hemodialysis is in decline both in the United States and worldwide. In the US less than 2% of dialysis patients are treated in this way. Throughout the world, the percentage of end stage renal disease patients on this therapy varies from less than 0.2% in Japan to 21.3% in Australia. Possible non-medical factors for this decline are discussed. Comparisons between dialysis therapies for survival, rehabilitation and cost are given. Finally, potential ways of increasing the number of patients being treated by this therapy are discussed.

References

1. Merrill JP, Schupack E, Cameron E. Hemodialysis in the home. JAMA 1964; 190: 468–70.

2. Curtis FK, Cole JJ, Fellow BJ, Tyler LL, Scribner BH. Hemodialysis in the home. Proc Eur Dialy Transpl Assoc 1965; 2: 99–101.
3. Delano BG, Feinroth MV, Feinroth M, Friedman EA, Home and medical center hemodialysis. Dollar comparison and payback period. JAMA 1981; 246: 230–232.
4. Tousignant P, Guttmann RD, Hollomby DJ. Transplantation and home hemodialysis: their cost-effectiveness. J Chronic Dis 1985; 38: 589–601.
5. Delano BG. The failure of home hemodialysis. Trans Am Soc Artif Intern Organs 1987; 33: 1–3.
6. US Renal Data Systems, USRDS 1993 Annual Data Report. The National Inst of Health. NIDDKD Bethesda Md Feb. 1993
7. Nissenson AR, Prichard SS, Ignatius KP, et al. Non-medical factors that impact on ESRD modality selection. Kidney Int 1993; 43: 120–127.
8. Mattern WD, McGaghie WC, Rigby RJ, Nissenson AR, Dunham CB, Khayrallah MA. Selection of ESRD treatment: An international study. Amer J Kidney Dis 1989; 13: 457–464.
9. HCFA releases 1991 End-Stage Renal Disease Program Data. Nephrology News & Issues 1993; 7: 13.
10. Blagg C. Home hemodialysis: A view from Seattle. Nephrology News & Issues 1992; 6: 33–36.
11. Inoue R. Automated Peritoneal Dialysis. The latest trend for dialysis patients? Contemporary Dialysis & Nephrology 1992; 13: 12.
12. DePaolo B, Cappelli P, Terenzio MG, et al. CAPD in the elderly: a 6-year experience. In: Ota K, Maher J, Winchester J Hirszel P, editors. Current concepts in peritoneal dialysis. New York: Excerta Medica, 1992, 667–669.
13. Rubin J, Hsu H, Bower J. Survival on Dialysis Therapy: One center's experience. Amer J Med Sci 1989; 297: 80–87.
14. Mailloux LU, Bellucci AG, Mossey RT, et al. Predictors of survival in patients undergoing dialysis. Amer J Med 1988; 84: 855–861.
15. Delano BG, Friedman EA. Correlates of decade-long technique survival on home hemodialysis. Trans Amer Soc Intern Organs 1990; 36: 337–339.
16. Gokal R. Quality of life in patients undergoing renal replacement therapy. Kidney Int 1993; 40: 523–27.
17. Evans RW. Recombinant Human Erythropoietin and the quality of life of end stage renal disease patients: A comparative analysis. Amer J Kidney Dis 1991; 18: 62–70.
18. Bremer BA McCauley CR, Wrona RM, Johnson JP. Quality of life in end-stage renal disease: A reexamination. Amer J Kidney Dis 1989; 13: 200–209.
19. Rubin J, Case G, Bower J. Comparison of rehabilitation in patients undergoing home dialysis. Continuous ambulatory or cyclic peritoneal dialysis vs home hemodialysis. Arch Intern Med 1990; 150: 1429–1431.
20. Inglehart JK. The American Health Care system. The end stage renal disease program. New Engl J Med 1993; 238: 366–371.
21. Croxson MComm BE, Ashton MA. A cost effectiveness analysis of the treatment of end stage renal failure. New Zealand Med J 1990; 103: 171–174.
22. Blagg CR. The challenge of hemodialysis. Contemporary Dialysis and Nephrology 1993; 14: 29–32.
23. Oberley ET, Leva R, Jorgensen L. Reflections on home hemodialysis: The invisible modality. Nephrology News & Issues 1992; 6: 24–29.

CHAPTER 18

Noncompliance frustrates formulae in maintenance dialysis patients

T.K. SREEPADA RAO, ANN SEALEY and ELI A. FRIEDMAN

Introduction

The leading causes of morbidity and mortality in patients with end stage renal disease (ESRD) who are treated by maintenance dialysis include cardiovascular diseases, renal osteodystrophy, infections (vascular access related and other systemic), and inadequate dialysis delivery. Many recent publications have focused on these issues, demonstrated various parameters to identify indices for poor patient survival, and have outlined steps to reduce morbidity and mortality [1–6]. One issue which has not received much attention is the role of, or lack thereof, patient's participation in his own care, and adherence to prescribed treatment regimen, in contributing to morbidity and mortality. Many urban dialysis centers are obliged to care for an increasing number of patients with renal failure who are intravenous drug addicts (IVDA), infected with the Human immunodeficiency virus (HIV), prisoners, undocumented aliens, homeless individuals, indigent patients with little or no family support. In such a clinical setting, noncompliance to prescribed therapy due to a variety of reasons is another major factor in limiting the ability of nephrologists to achieve the goals of renal replacement therapy in ESRD subjects.

Kings County Hospital Center, one of the largest municipal health care facilities in the US, provides dialysis care in Brooklyn, NY, for patients with ESRD who are largely poor, uninsured, homeless, prisoners, and many are undocumented aliens. A majority of patients evaluated by the renal physicians have little or no knowledge of kidney disease, and have reached ESRD by the time of their first encounter with the health team in the emergency room. Many are acutely ill with severe uremia, gross fluid overload, and hyperkalemia, requiring emergency dialysis support when seen initially. After the primary rescue treatments, the reality of irreversible nature of their renal disease, the need for life long therapy, and adjustments to a new restrictive life style of dialysis and dietary restrictions, is extremely difficult, if not impossible, for many patients to accept. The renal health care team faces an uphill

E. A. Friedman (ed.), Death on Hemodialysis, 183–188.
© 1994 *Kluwer Academic Publishers.*

Table 1. Causes of new onset ESRD in 1992

	n = 76		
1.	Hypertension	26	(33%)
2.	Diabetes Mellitus	16	(21%)
3.	HIV Associated Nephropathy	15	(20%)
4.	Chronic Glomerulonephritis	10	(13%)
5.	Systemic Lupus Erythematosus	3	(4%)
6.	Sickle cell Nephropathy	2	(3%)
7.	Obstructive Nephropathy	2	(3%)
8.	Polycystic Kidney disease	1	(1.5%)
9.	Multiple Myeloma	1	(1.5%)

ESRD = End stage renal disease
HIV = Human immunodeficiency virus

task in educating patients, enlisting compliance both acutely during the initial hospitalization (such as vascular access surgery, femoral vein catheterization for hemodialysis, renal biopsy etc.), and subsequently during outpatient ambulatory dialysis therapy. Patient education about the advantages and disadvantages of different modalities of renal replacement therapy, and a truly informed option by consumers in choosing the type of maintenance dialysis, or renal transplantation is not a reality for many. This communication will attempt to address some aspects of patient noncompliance in ESRD patients during the initial hospitalization, and subsequently while receiving maintenance hemodialysis in an urban facility.

Materials, methods, and results

From January 1, 1992 through December 31, 1992, maintenance hemodialysis was started in 76 patients who were admitted to Kings County Hospital with new onset ESRD. The presumed renal diagnoses in these patients are listed in Table 1. HIV associated nephropathy accounted for 15 (20%) of ESRD, 9 of whom were IVDA. Only 5 of the 76 patients (6%) were electively admitted to the hospital with a functioning arterio-venous access for the initiation of hemodialysis. In two patients, vascular access had been performed in a foreign country, in another Brooklyn facility in one, and at our institution in only two subjects. 56 of the 76 patients (74%), were either unaware of kidney problems in the past, or had very little understanding of renal disease at the time of initial evaluation by the admitting physicians in the emergency room. The difficulties experienced by the renal team in the management of one such poorly informed, psychopathic patient are illustrated below.

C.T., 30 yrs old unemployed black man, an IVDA and HIV seropositive was admitted on 8/12/92 with nephrotic syndrome secondary to HIVAN, with an endogenous Ccr of 9 ml/min. After detailed discussion, and several 'education' sessions with the patient, he could not be convinced to undergo an elective vascular access surgery, or apply for medical assistance. He was discharged from the hospital three weeks later with a clinic appointment for follow-up care. Patient was readmitted in December 1992 with further worsening of renal function. He seemed receptive to physician's recommendation, but signed against medical advice on the day of scheduled access surgery. He was again admitted in January 93 with severe uremia, serum potassium of 8.5 meq/l, and an emergency hemodialysis was performed in the emergency room employing femoral vein catheterization. Over the next 3 weeks he refused all access procedures, and agreed to undergo femoral vein hemodialysis intermittently off and on. Over the next 8 weeks vascular access surgery could not be performed because of patient's refusal, his disappearance from the hospital on the day of surgery without staff permission, and his refusal of pre operative hemodialysis, or blood transfusions. When he finally consented, access procedure had to be postponed on 4 occasions because of development of fever on the morning of surgery. Since these episodes were sporadic, and no etiology could be found, the staff felt that fever was self induced by the patient presumably because of his not wanting to be discharged from the comforts of a hospital to a shelter. During this period, hemodialysis was being intermittently accomplished via repeated femoral vein catheters, many occasions as an emergency (disrupting the schedule of physicians and nurses) due either to hyperkalemia or pulmonary edema. Finally, for fear of administrative actions, he agreed to a permacath insertion, which was carried out on 3/20/93, and was discharged from the hospital on 3/25/93. The patient returned for outpatient hemodialysis only once the following week, and could not be reached because of wrong reported address. He was brought in by the emergency medical service on 4/12/93 with extreme weakness, lethargy, hypotension, gross fluid overload, and a hematocrit of 12%. The patient could not be hemodialyzed because of hemodynamic instability (BP 60/40) despite blood transfusions and colloid infusions, and expired on 4/14/93.

To assess noncompliance in ambulatory subjects, the medical records of all 106 patients (many started on dialysis prior to 1992) who underwent outpatient maintenance hemodialysis for 2 months or more in the calendar year 1992 were reviewed. For the purposes of this study, noncompliance was defined as missing two or more scheduled hemodialysis treatments in a month for two months or more. Demographic data of noncompliant patients was compared with those who were compliant to the prescribed regimen. 21 of 106 patients (21%) were noncompliant by the above definition, 9 of whom missed treatments more than twice a month for 4 months or more. No significant differences in the age, sex, and renal diagnosis could be ascertained between the compliant and noncompliant groups. There were 40 deaths in maintenance hemodialysis patients in 1992. The causes of death in 9 of these 40 patients (22%) were hyperkalemia in 3, pulmonary edema in 3, and unknown (found dead at home) in the remaining 3, all attributable directly or indirectly to patient's noncompliance. AIDS related complications led to death in 20 patients (50%), and homicide was the cause in 2 others.

Discussion

The modern management of chronic renal insufficiency consists of developing an individualized life plan for each patient depending on the age, medical status, co-morbid conditions, family support, availability of living organ donors, and financial resources for long term care. The preparation of patients for the inevitable reality of ESRD should start early, once a diagnosis of chronic renal failure is established. A key component of care is the education of patients and the family about ESRD with an emphasis on the lifelong nature of the illness, and the need for active participation by both parties during a prolonged course of supervised medical care. This will greatly facilitate a knowledgeable patient to make decisions about the choice of renal replacement therapy and adhere to the regimen. The preferred time for education is while patients with residual renal function are still being managed conservatively. Depending upon medical criterian, and personal preferences, patients/family in conjunction with the nephrologist should choose either hemodialysis, peritoneal dialysis or renal transplantation. With a well-informed patient, compliance to prescribed therapy is readily accomplished, and efforts can now be focused on the best possible use of limited available resources in electively preparing patients to receive maintenance dialysis or renal transplantation, to achieve maximum rehabilitation, and to minimize subsequent morbidity and mortality.

Inner city renal care centers such as ours which treat a large number of ESRD patients who are indigent with no family physician, medically least informed, and with little family support for coping with chronic illnesses, are frustrated by their inability to provide elective and optimal care because of budgetary constraints and patient's reluctance to follow recommendations. In addition, IVDA with self-destructive personalities, prisoners, homeless persons who miss treatment schedules and are repeatedly brought to the emergency rooms requiring urgent care, not only are deranging the smooth functioning of dialysis units thus compromising care to compliant patients, but also are a constant drain on other hospital resources as well. Many undocumented aliens are ineligible for federally funded health benefits, and renal transplantation may not be feasible even in ideal candidates. Because of fear of deportation, many aliens refuse to provide personal details further complicating our ability to reach out when treatments are missed or scheduled consultant clinic appointments are not kept. Also, some HIV patients, cognizant of the incurable nature of their infection, are further reluctant to accept and adopt to ESRD, another irreversible illness. All these factors complicate the process of both patient education in electively planning renal therapy during their initial hospitalization, and subsequently during ambulatory dialysis care. Data obtained for 1992 alone at our institution revealed that a majority are uneducated and uninformed about renal failure at the time of diagnosis, and elective start of maintenance dialysis therapy is an unachievable goal. The irreversible, and lifelong nature of the renal illness contributes further to the unwillingness in accepting the reality, and frustrates our ability to achieve compliance from patients to undergo surgical procedures. Prolonged patient hospitalization resulting from nonacceptance and noncompliance adds greatly to the economic burden of renal failure therapy. The case report illustrated above underscores these issues, highlights our inability to provide care serve as and an example of wastage of enormous time and resources consequent to noncompliance.

The US Renal Data Systems report, and other studies, have indicated that mortality rates in dialysis patients in the US are higher than those observed in other industrialized nations [1–2]. Inadequate dialysis delivery, either due to shortened dialysis time or because of reuse of hemodialyzers, is one of the major reasons cited to explain these findings [3–5]. From the observations made in our center, patient noncompliance, a factor which has received less attention in the past, also contributes significantly to poor dialysis care and an increase in morbidity and mortality. The 21% noncompliance rate in our ambulatory patients is unacceptably high, and its impact on disrupting the efficient functioning of dialysis units is enormous in terms of economic loss and personnel morale. Although no demographic differences were seen between the compliant and noncompliant group, many patients who missed prescribed therapy were either IVDA, or homeless individuals, or those with little family support. Clearly, inadequate dialysis resulted in hyperkalemia, and fluid overload contributing to a high mortality in these patients.

In the past, we and others have reported that despite adequate dialysis and nutritional support, the survival of patients with AIDS and ESRD treated by maintenance hemodialysis is very poor [7–9]. In 1992, 20 of 40 (50%) deaths in our center was attributable to AIDS, even though a majority were compliant, received erythropoietin, and adequate dialysis [10], indicating our inability to improve prognosis in this subset of patients. While deaths due to AIDS may be inevitable at our present level of knowledge, homicides beyond control in our patients, noncompliance to therapy is clearly a modifiable risk factor. In brief, in large cities noncompliance not only frustrates efficient treatment formulae, but also contributes greatly to morbidity and mortality. There is a great need to enhance efforts to educate the public about health disorders in minorities, problems of drug abuse, and HIV infection, with an emphasis on preventive aspects. Unfortunately, federal budget cutbacks and health care reforms in the US have contributed to these problems, and unless adequate steps are taken to change the directions, these undesirable trends are likely to continue.

References

1. Held PJ, Brunner F, Odaka M, Garcia J, Port FK, Gaylin DS. Five year survival for end stage renal disease patients in the US, Europe, and Japan 1982–87. Am J Kidney Dis 1990; 15: 451–457.
2. US Renal Data System: USRDS 1991 Annual Data Report. Am J Kidney Dis 1991; 18 (Suppl 2): 1–127.

3. Held PJ, Blagg CR, Liska DW, Port FK, Hakim R, Levin NW. Adequacy of hemodialysis according to dialysis prescription in Europe and the United States. Kidney Int 1992; 42 (Suppl 38): S16–S21.
4. Held PJ, Levin NW, Bovbjerg RR, Pauly MV, Diamond LH. Mortality and duration of hemodialysis treatment. JAMA 1991; 265: 871–875.
5. Vanholder R, Ringoir S. Infectious morbidity and defects of phagocytic function in end stage renal disease: a review. J Am Soc Nephrol 1993; 3: 1541–1554.
6. Goldwasser P, Mittman N, Antignani A, Burrell D, Michel MA, Collier J, Avram MM. Predictors of mortality in hemodialysis patients. J Am Soc Nephrol 1993; 3: 1613–1622.
7. Rao TKS. Maintenance dialysis in patients with Human immunodeficiency virus infection. Seminars in Dialysis. 1988; 1(4): 203–208.
8. Ortiz C, Meneses R, Jaffe JA Fernandez JA, Perez G, Bourgoignie JJ. Outcome of patients with Human immunodeficiency virus on maintenance hemodialysis. Kidney Int 1988; 34: 248–253.
9. Feinfeld DA, Kaplan R, Dressler R, Lynn I. Survival of human immunodeficiency virus-infected patients on maintenance dialysis. Clin Nephrol 1989; 32(5): 221–224.
10. Shrivastava D, Rao TKS, Lundin P, Sealey A, Friedman, EA. Erythropoietin is efficacious in patients with end stage renal disease and human immunodeficiency virus infection. J Am Soc Nephrol 1992; 3(3): 431.

CHAPTER 19

The UK dialysis picture revisited

GEOFFREY M. BERLYNE

Introduction

In 1982, I published an editorial in Nephron, 'Over 50 + Uremic = Death', to draw attention to the failure of the British National Health Service to provide dialysis services for the over middle aged and to those suffering from extra-renal disease [1]. This resulted in anger against the messenger: first there was a stage of denial, then later acceptance that all was not well, and then some correction of the situation [2–4].

By 1985, I followed with a second editorial [5] pointing out some improvement, largely due to the nephrologists in the UK. Nevertheless, my anxiety for the untreated, neglected renal failure patient condemned to death in a deadly bureaucratic system in the UK was described as 'emotional' and even in 1990 [6] it was suggested that they needed to cut up the cake of available health service money carefully depending on the various competing requirements as a justification for the foot dragging. Shades of Relman. I still believe I needed to bat for the dialysis patients being denied therapy. Nevertheless, my initial shattering of equanimity in 1982 has had some effect, and indeed in one 1990 paper, in which Mallick was the moving figure, it was pointed out that even the approximate 60/million new patients per annum was inadequate and more likely 80/million need treating in the UK [7].

What is the situation at the moment? How much unremicide is there?

The tables for 1991 and 1990 are now available from the EDTA registry and Mallick has been kind enough to obtain breakdowns of the age groups in the UK on dialysis for 1990.

You will see in Table 1:
1) That the overall number of new patients on various forms of dialysis has tripled from 1982 to 1991 from 19.9 to 60.7 per million, and that is no mean feat, but it is somewhat below the European mean.
2) That the number of older persons (over 55) has grown considerably both on hemodialysis and on peritoneal dialysis so that it is *no longer true* that

189

E. A. Friedman (ed.), Death on Hemodialysis, 189–194.
© 1994 *Kluwer Academic Publishers.*

Table 1. Number of patients (per million population) accepted for dialysis each year in European countries.

	1982	1988	1990	1991
Austria	38.1	95.7	101	105.3
Belgium	39.6	85.2	96.7	86.7
Israel	58.2	80.0	114.7	106.3
Federal Republic of Germany	44.0	77.0	79.2	94.1
Holland	27.4	65.3	68.5	60.0
Sweden	41.3	64.3	66.3	99.6
Switzerland	44.5	61.8	76.9	95.5
Greece	18.8	59.2	75.4	70.6
Spain	32.7	57.1	59.8	59.5
France	30.9	56.3	56.5	77.1
United Kingdom	19.9	55.1	60.7	59.7
Italy	65.0	86.0	89.0	53.9
Norway	37.3	52.7	67.1	65.3
Denmark	26.9	52.5	51.8	47.5
Ireland	19.4	33.8	42.4	48.2
Mean	36.26	65.47	73.73	75.29
SD	13.470	16.30	19.78	20.98
Median	37.3	61.8	68.5	70.6

Table 2. Breakdown for age of new patients on dialysis in year 1985–1990 (supplied by courtesy of Dr. N. Mallick).

New patients on dialysis each year

Year	1985	1986	1987	1988	1989	1990
Total number	2285	2385	2272	2114	1899	1432
Over 55 years	996	1106	1077	1029	962	789
% of total who are > 55 years	43.6	46.4	47.4	48.7	50.7	55.1

over 50 and uremia = death in the UK. (Tables 2, 6). Wing has illustrated this in detail [2].

3) There are insufficient nephrologists (1.5 full time equivalent per million) and insufficient renal units in the UK, so the renal units are massive and the nephrologists have a huge burden of patients. This is either a deliberate step for no apparent reason or more likely, a bureaucratic screw up of immense proportions. I favor the latter; muddling through is a well known British talent and unfortunately often remains a 'muddle'.

To counter the statement that funds do not permit, let us look at financial data from the World Bank [1] about European Countries covered by the EDTA registry for the year 1990 (Table 3). We are restricted to 1990 because the World Bank data so far released do not go beyond 1990. The GNP is compared to the numbers of new patients/million put on dialysis for 1990 in Europe. The UK is in the upper half of the GNP, but at just over $16,000 per

Table 3. Ranking of GNP per capita and by number of patients taken on dialysis the first for 20 European countries. US data given for comparison but not taken into statistical analysis.

Ranking of new patients/year/million by country for 1990		Ranking of GNP/capita	GNP/capita by country for 1990
Austria	101.1	Switzerland	$ 32,680
Belgium	96.7	Finland	26,040
W. Germany	79.2	Sweden	23,660
Switzerland	76.9	Norway	23,120
Greece	75.4	W. Germany	22,230
Portugal	74.7	France	19.490
Netherland	68.5	Austria	19,060
Norway	67.1	Netherland	17,320
Sweden	66.3	Italy	16,830
UK	60.7	UK	16,100
Spain	59.8	Belgium	15,540
France	56.5	Spain	11,020
Denmark	51.8	Ireland	9,540
Italy	50.0	Greece	5,990
Finland	49.3	Portugal	4,900
Czechoslovakia	46.3	Czechoslovakia	3,140
Yugoslavia	44.4	Yugoslavia	3,060
Ireland	42.4	Hungary	2,780
Bulgaria	40.4	Poland	1,690
Poland	19.3	Romania	1,640
US (1989)	166.0	US	21,790
Mean of 20 (excl. US) pts/million	65	Mean GNP (excl. US)	$13,792
		Semi	2091.517
SD	22.33568	SD	9353.548
Median	63.5	Median	15,820

year, not as high as France, Italy, Austria, Denmark, Finland or Switzerland in Europe. The US has a GNP under $22,000 but had 166 new patients/million. Japan had both a higher GNP and about 150 new patients/million. Belgium, Austria and West Germany were ahead a little in recruitment. So in summary, the UK had in 1990 intakes similar to the leading European countries but less than some (West Germany, Belgium, Austria, Greece and Portugal) – the latter 2 are of interest because of their profound poverty in European terms – GNP <$7,000 per capita – yet managing to put more patients on dialysis than richer countries in Europe such as the UK. If we look at GNP/million population factored by new patients per million (Table 4) we see that the UK has a sum of $256.6 $\times$ 10^6/new dialysis patient, i.e. close to that of Germany ($280.7 $\times$ 10^6) but Portugal has only $65.6 $\times$ 10^6, Belgium $160.7 $\times$ 10^6, Greece $79 $\times$ 10^6. The US has $153.2 $\times$ 10^6 and Japan $169.5 $\times$ 10^6. These tables indicate that a greater slice of the larger GNP in the US and Japan, and of the smaller GNP in Belgium, Greece, Spain and Portugal is going to put

Table 4. Shows data for 1990. Includes government spending on health care as a percentage of government income, number of new patients/million and GNP per million/number of new patients per million. Countries where some 1990 data are absent from World Bank tables are excluded e.g. Switzerland

	% Health care	# New patient/million	$ (GNP/new patient)
Austria	12.9	101.1	188.6
Belgium	4.1	40.4	160.7
Czechoslovakia	0.4	46.3	67.8
Denmark	1.1	51.8	426.3
Finland	10.8	49.3	528.2
France	15.2	56.5	345
W. Germany	19.3	79.2	280.7
Hungary	7.9	41.6	66.8
Ireland	12.1	42.4	252.2
Italy	11.3	50	336.6
Netherland	11.7	68.5	252.9
Poland	10.4	19.3	344.6
Spain	12.8	59.8	184.2
Sweden	0.9	66.3	356.9
UK	14.6	60.7	265.2
USA	13.5	166	153.2

new patients on dialysis. This is a decision in each country and is presumably decided by:

1) Political pressures/expediency
2) Power of MD and patient lobbies in democracies
3) Degree of control of bureaucrats who are not primarily imbued with a sense of devotion to the patients' welfare in any country.

Table 3 shows the number of new patients/million for 20 European Countries ranked from highest to lowest in 1990. The mean is 65.1, median 63.5; the UK falls just short at 60.7. In GNP, ranked from highest to lowest, mean is $13.792, median is $15.820.00. The UK falls a little above the median. Thus, in European terms, the UK has an average intake. In 1990 there was some short fall-off of new patients in the UK both below and above 55 years old.

Contrary to what may have been implied, the increased intake in the UK has not been due to mostly using CAPD, but has been due to fairly even allocation to both peritoneal and hemodialysis. Indeed, Table 5 shows that hemodialysis has a slight edge in the elderly.

A major problem has been shown to be lack of referral of suitable cases in the UK to nephrologists. This prompted some of the mindless statements against my 1982 editorial in the vein that 'there is no shortage – we dialyze all the cases referred to us that are suitable'. The problem still exists 13 years later, i.e. that GP's and consultants in medicine are still not referring perhaps half of the patients who could benefit from, particularly in the elderly.

Moreover, the questionnaire of Challah and colleagues [12] showed the attitude to dialysis of consultant physicians and GP's who demonstrated not

Table 5. Shows distribution of CAPD and HD in new patients coming into dialysis in each of years 1985 through 1990. Transplantations not included (supplied courtesy of Dr. N. Mallick).

Year	1985	1986	1987	1988	1989	1990
HD (Under 55)	641	605	651	555	441	354
(Over 55)	482	560	540	531	548	504
CAPD/IPD (Under 55)	447	501	445	491	448	296
(Over 55)	507	539	532	511	409	282
Total CAPD + HD (< 55)	1088	1106	1096	1046	889	650
(> 55)	989	1099	1072	1042	957	786
% CAPD total dialysis						
patients (< 55)	41.1	45.3	40.6	46.9	50.4	45.5
(> 55)	51.3	49.0	49.6	49.0	42.7	35.9

only ignorance and prejudice, but, surprisingly, some peculiar attitudes of nephrologists, 45% of whom rejected a 50 year old man with ischemic heart disease; 79.1% rejected a 52 year old alcoholic and 86.8% of nephrologists rejected a 29 year old hepatitis B positive man. In the US, this would be actionable.

Trousseau would turn over in his grave – 'guerir quelquefois, soulager souvent, consoler toujours'. However, this study was published in 1984 and it is likely that attitudes have changed. At least I hope so.

How do we explain the discrepancy between what the UK nephrologists consider to be a reasonable demand goal for dialysis at 80 new patients/million, and the US/Japanese numbers of taking 160 per million, Israel 114.7, Austria 101.1 and Belgium's 96.7/million?

The answer may be in the following:

1) The UK nephrologists are aiming too low (as the questionnaire of Challah *et al* would suggest), and they are too pessimistic about the results.
2) In the US, Japan, Italy, Austria and Belgium, nephrologists are putting on too many patients, possibly for venal reasons.
3) Varying incidence of renal failure in different countries – eg. stone disease in Italy and the US; HIV nephropathy in the US; diabetic glomerulopathy in the US as a cause of 1/3 all ESRD new patients. This may cause a greater load of patients outside the UK.

Unfortunately, I have insufficient data to decide if any of these is correct; perhaps all 3 are, perhaps none are.

Conclusion

The position of dialysis in the UK has improved. The number of older patients has increased considerably. There is still some way to go before the modest target of 80 new patients per million is achieved. There is a profound shortage of renal consultants and units which needs a solution, and the UK government needs to sort this out, but then they have a lot of sorting out of priorities to do. So does the US government.

The basic problems of a NHS financial cake cut in an unacceptable manner from the point of view of nephrologists and the need for education of the GP's, internists, and nephrologists need to be highlighted. The nephrologists should continue to rock the boat, so as to achieve a greater chance of survival for their patients.

Acknowledgements

I wish to thank Dr. Netar Mallick, Chairman of the EDTA Registry, for supplying data on the age groups and types of dialysis in the United Kingdom from 1985–1990.

References

1. Berlyne GM. Over 50 + Uremic x Death. Nephron 1982; 31: 189–190.
2. Wing AJ. A different view from different countries: United Kingdom. In: CM Kjellstrand and JB Dossetor, editors. Ethical problems in dialysis and transplantation. Kluwer, Boston, 1992; 201–226.
3. Halper T. The misfortunes of others: end-stage renal failure in the United Kingdom. Cambridge University Press, 1989.
4. Nissenson AR, Richard SS, Cheng IKP, et al. Non-medical factors that impact on ESRD modalilty selection. Kidney International 1993; (43)40: S120–127.
5. Berlyne GM. The British dialysis tragedy revisited. Nephron 1985; 41: 305–306.
6. McGown MG. The prevalence of advanced renal failure in Northern Ireland. British Medical Journal 1990; 301: 900–903.
7. Feest TG, Mistry CD, Grimas DS, Mallick NP. Incidence of advanced chronic renal failure in the United Kingdom and the need for end-stage renal replacement treatment. British Medical Journal 1990; 301: 897–900.
8. Wing AJ. Renal Replacement therapy-too little or too much? In: Raine AG. Advanced Renal Medicine. Oxford: Oxford University Press, 1992; 465–475.
9. Wing AJ. Can we meet the real need for dialysis and transplantation? (Editorial). British Medical Journal 1990; (301): 885–886.
10. EDTA. Combined report on regular dialysis and transplantation in Europe XXI 1990. Nephrology Dialysis Transplantation 1991; (6)4: 6.
11. World Bank World Development Report. Development and the Environment. New York: Oxford University Press, 1992; 227.
12. Challah S, Wing AJ, Bauer R, et al. Negative selection of patients for dialysis and transplantation in the United Kingdom. British Medical Journal 1984; 288: 111–129.

CHAPTER 20

Blood pressure control: the neglected factor that affects survival of dialysis patients

BELDING H. SCRIBNER

There are four major factors that affect survival of dialysis patients. They are: 1) the dose of dialysis 2) protein and calorie intake 3) smoking and 4) control of blood pressure. In the current dialysis literature most publications deal extensively with the dose of dialysis and to a somewhat lesser extent, the nutrition of the patient. In contrast, virtually no current meetings or publications deal with the ill effects of smoking and hypertension as risk factors that have a strong adverse effect on the survival of dialysis patients. Two examples: a review of the table of contents of this volume will reveal that the topic is not addressed in a separate presentation; a supplement to the Feb. 1993 issue of Kidney International contained 15 manuscripts from an excellent international meeting comparing the results of hemodialysis and peritoneal dialysis. None of the manuscripts dealt with the subject of control of hypertension.

Ever since the original observations of Haire and Sherrard et al. [1] and of Lundin et al. [2] back in the late 1970's, it has been clearly established that in the dialysis population, hypertension is associated with the lethal complications of accelerated atherosclerosis. However, it remained for Charra et al. [3] to demonstrate that control of hypertension could prevent these complications. Perhaps it was the fact that their 1983 paper [3] did not attract the attention it should have, that caused most nephrologists to neglect control of hypertension in their publications. However Charra's landmark publication in 1992 [4] presents convincingly the best patient survival data so far published. This excellent paper together with a follow up editorial by Charra [5], firmly establishes control of hypertension as the major reason for their excellent survival results. These important publications clearly make it mandatory that control of blood pressure must become an integral part of the care of the patient on dialysis.

Control of blood pressure among dialysis patients presents certain serious difficulties, which may further explain why the subject is avoided. These difficulties include the following: 1) time on dialysis may have to be prolonged; 2) antihypertensive medications cause serious side effects, especially severe

195

E. A. Friedman (ed.), Death on Hemodialysis, 195–197.
© 1994 *Kluwer Academic Publishers.*

hypotension during fluid removal; 3) Compliance with the 3–4 gram sodium diet is often a problem. Charra *et al.* [3,4] easily solve these problems because they use old fashioned Kiil dialyzers and dialyze 8 hours per session. This slow gentle dialysis technic permits them to use aggressive ultrafiltration to reduce the size of the extracellular volume to the point where no antihypertensive medications are needed in 98% of their 445 patients [4]. The question remains: Is it possible to use modern high efficiency dialysis equipment and still achieve good blood pressure control?

Before I attempt to answer that question, let me present an historical vignette. Back in the spring of 1960, our first patient, Clyde Shields, was dying of malignant hypertension. What few drugs were then available were totally ineffective. We decided that the only chance we had to save Clyde was to reduce his extracellular volume to the point where he had to drop his blood pressure. It took about three months of aggressive ultrafiltration during each dialysis to gradually bring his blood pressure under control. These sessions often were complicated by severe cramping and sudden hypotension. However, once he became normotensive, he remained so for the next 11 years of his life. This sequence was repeated on several other patients during the early years. However, it was Laurent and Charra in Tassin that perfected the method of blood pressure control. As described by Charra *et al.* [4] when a new patient is started on dialysis in Tassin, much the same sequence is followed. Using aggressive ultrafiltration, they gradually withdraw all antihypertensive medications. This process may take from 2 to 6 months and is called the *transition* phase. Reducing the sodium intake as low as possible during the transition phase reduces the incidence and severity of the hypotensive episodes. This transition phase demands patience and persistence on the part of the nephrologist, and willingness to tolerate some cramping and hypotension on the part of the patient. Once the patient is normotensive off antihypertensive medications, sodium intake can be liberalized to the 3–6 gram range depending on the patient's tolerance to ultrafiltration during hemodialysis.

Now to answer the above question. I believe that any nephrologist can duplicate Charra's results using any kind of equipment just so long as he or she understands the process, particularly the difficulties to expect during the transition phase. Also there may be other approaches to the control of blood pressure in hemodialysis patients; but publication is lacking.

In theory, starting a patient on CAPD instead of hemodialysis should avoid the difficult transition phase. With CAPD, fluid removal is both constant and relatively easy to control. Therefore the wide swings in extracellular volume inherent in the 3 x weekly hemodialysis cycle do not occur. Hence it should be much easier to lower the volume of the extracellular space to the point where antihypertensive medications can be stopped. A recent publication [6] provides preliminary verification of this prediction. Saldahna *et al.* [6] have shown in a series of patients on CAPD that a higher percentage are off antihypertensive medications and the average blood pressure is lower than in a comparable group of hemodialysis patients.

Finally, it is worth pointing out that control of blood pressure *must* begin when loss of kidney function first is diagnosed. We have long maintained that control of blood pressure is the single most important factor in slowing the progression of kidney disease to end stage [7–10]. An important study which strongly supports this point of view recently has been publised [11].

In conclusion, because of the spectacular survival results achieved by Charra *et al* [4,5], it now becomes incumbent on all nephrologists to devise methods of normalizing the blood pressure of their dialysis patients.

References

1. Haire HM, Sherrard DJ, Scarpadane D, Curtis FK, Brunzell JD. Smoking, hypertension and mortality in a maintenance dialysis population. Cardiovasc Med 1978; 3: 1163–1168.
2. Lundin AP, Adler, AJ, Feinroth MV, Berlyne GM, Friedman EA. Maintenance dialysis. Survival beyond the first decade. JAMA 1980; 244: 38–40.
3. Charra B, Calemard E, Laurent G. Control of hypertension and prolonged survival on maintenance hemodialysis. Nephron 1983; 33: 96–99.
4. Charra B, Calemard E, Ruffet M, Chazot C, Terrat JC, Vanel T, Laurent G. Survival as an index of adequacy of dialysis. Kidney Int 1992; 41: 1286–1291.
5. Charra, B. Editorial: Does emperical long slow dialysis improve survival on dialysis? If so, how and why? (In press).
6. Saldanha LF, Weiler EWJ, Gonick HC. Effect of continuous ambulatory peritoneal dialysis on blood pressure control. Am J Kidney Dis 1993; 21: 184–188.
7. Scribner BH, Fergus EB, Boen ST, Thomas ED. Some therapeutic approaches to chronic renal insufficiency. Ann Rev Med 1965; 16: 285–300.
8. Ulvila JM, Kennedy JA, Lamberg JD, Scribner BH. Blood pressure in chronic renal failure: Effect of sodium intake and furosemide. J Am Med Assoc 1972; 220: 233–238.
9. Davidson RC, Scribner BH. Basil sodium excretion in the treatment of hypertension in chronic renal disease. Cardiovasc Med 1976; 1: 259–264.
10. Scribner BH. Salt and hypertension. J Am Med Assoc 1983; 250: 388–389.
11. Walker WG, Neaton JD, Cutler JA, Neuworth R, Cohen JD. Renal function change in hypertensive members of the multiple risk factor intervention trial. J Am Med Assoc 1992; 268: 3085–3091.

CHAPTER 21

Many deaths in hemodialysis patients are preventable

A. PETER LUNDIN

Introduction

Preventable deaths occur in every medical practice. These events are always regrettable but are an inevitable measure of the imperfection of medicine and its practioners. In the case of hemodialysis patients, however, available evidence would suggest that the number of preventable deaths exceeds the inevitable. So great is the problem, I believe, that if its full extent were revealed, the situation would be seen as a major scandal and a national tragedy.

Preventing deaths in hemodialysis patients

The excess mortality in hemodialysis patients compared with Japan and Europe [1], when examined in another perspective, indicates that a substantial number of these deaths could be prevented. Reduction of excess mortality as well as morbidity requires careful analysis of the reasons why patients die, followed by implementation of methods and procedures for the purpose of decreasing the incidence of these morbid and mortal events. In order to successfully reduce these adverse occurrences, contributing factors must be sought out and their impact reduced wherever possible. Last but not least, is the human factor: the skills, dedication and interest of those caring for dialysis patients. Absence of these qualities in dialysis professionals may have the most profoundly adverse effect of all.

Analysis of causes of death in hemodialysis patients

In most listings of causes of death, the majority are given to be cardiac problems and infections. In Europe, according to the European Dialysis and Transplant Association data for 1990, 65% of deaths were from these causes (Table 1) [2]. In a paper published in 1982 [3] that should be better known,

199

E. A. Friedman (ed.), Death on Hemodialysis, 199–204.
© 1994 *Kluwer Academic Publishers.*

Table 1. Causes of death in European hemodialysis patients, 1990

Cardiovascular	53%
– Myocardial ischemia, infarction	15%
– Cerebrovascular	11%
– Cardiac arrest	12%
– Cardiac failure	12%
– Other cardiac	3%
Infection	12%

Table 2. Possible etiologies listed under cardiac arrest, cardiac failure, other cardiac

Acute pulmonary edema
Hyperkalemia, other arrhythmia
Cardiomyopathy
Pericarditis

Plough and Salem point out the fallacy of accepting the accuracy of cause of death as listed in the Death Notification Form. In a careful review of the medical records of 24 hemodialysis patients among 40 total, whose deaths had been listed as cardiac related (60%), they found that only 5 (12.5%) were truly cardiac in nature. One third (8) were due to dietary indiscretion (a cause not originally listed) and another 5 were due to 'treatment related accidents'. Of the total of 40 deaths, those amenable to prevention include: 11 due to dietary indiscretion, 7 due to treatment related accidents (1 on original list), and 5 as result of septicemia and localized infections (pre AIDS), adding up to 23 of 40 (57.5%). Cause of death originally listed but not supported by chart review include: respiratory arrest (2), renal failure (2), embolism (2), and unknown (3).

Heart attacks and strokes in dialysis patients may be inevitable when due to certain preexisting conditions. For longer term patients with simple renal failure, death from cardiac ischemia and stroke may instead be the result of failure to control the blood pressure. Underdefined categories called cardiac arrest, cardiac failure and other cardiac as listed in the EDTA report are, in the main, likely to consist of potentially preventable causes (Table 2). Some patients may gain more than 7 to 8% of their body weight in fluid accumulated between dialysis treatments and present in acute pulmonary edema to the dialysis facility or hospital emergency room. Eventually they will do this one time too often, resulting in death. Such patients are not beyond redemption, however. I have known patients that would gain more than 20 lbs of water between their dialysis treatments, whose behavior was turned around by conflict resolution and the concern and patience of the staff. The same can be true for those at risk of arrhythmia and cardiac arrest from excess intake of potassium. It should be noted that potassium levels less than 8 are rarely fatal in a dialysis patient.

When a patient goes into pulmonary edema after gaining considerably less than what is usually considered dangerous, the problem is often due to a failure to bring him to his correct dry weight. Persistently catabolic or undernourished dialysis patients lose weight which may not be detected unless looked for by a rise in blood pressure, a drop in albumin or other markers of nutrition. Cardiomyopathy due to whatever cause is easily detectable by echocardiography and should not be assumed to be a cause of death unless diagnosed. Pericarditis, unless demonstrated to be viral in origin, is simply due to underdialysis [4].

Infection is another potentially preventable cause of death in hemodialysis patients. It has been amply demonstrated that, among severely immunodepressed AIDS patients, prophylaxis as well as early detection and treatment of some infections can prolong life. Hemodialysis patients, even when underdialyzed, are not so severely immunosuppressed that they develop infections with opportunistic organisms. The types of infections for which they are at risk are preventable by appropriate technique when related to the blood access. When infections involve other organ systems, they are often detectable early and are certainly treatable. It is in fact the failure to prevent infection, or to detect it early and treat it promptly, that is responsible for most of the infection related deaths in hemodialysis patients without AIDS.

Determining and correcting contributory factors

Underlying and exacerbating all the other problems besieging dialysis patients is the probability that many are being inadequately dialyzed. Underdialysis may, in fact, be the most important cause of death in dialysis patients, whether primary or in contributing to death from other illnesses. The patient who is inadequately dialyzed is being maintained in a symptomatically uremic state, manifesting uremic complications. Adequate dialysis, on the other hand, would be a level of efficiency that makes the patient asymptomatic and at little risk of recurrent uremic complications. Malnutrition due to poor appetite with loss of real weight is typical of uremia. A well dialyzed patient, who eats well and is without other medical problems, should not lose body tissue and will maintain or regain real weight because a good appetite will allow an adequate intake of protein and calories without the need for supplementation. Well dialyzed patients look well and feel good and are less susceptible to infection and resistant to uremic pericarditis. In fact their risk of death, certainly within the first 10 years of treatment, should not be much greater than that of age and disease matched cohorts.

Sadly, the reality is quite different for many dialysis patients. Over the years when skilled practioners of the art and science of hemodialysis conversed informally, they often arrived at a consensus that many patients were likely to be poorly dialyzed. More concretely, Held et al using data from the USRDS have shown that many American patients are dialyzed at an efficiency below that shown to be satisfactory [5]. When added to evidence that the death rate for dialysis patients in the United States is higher than that in Europe and Japan, it is hard to avoid the conclusion that underdialysis is a major primary or contributory cause of death for dialysis patients in this country. And if that is the case, then many of these deaths are preventable.

Some blame may go to the government because of failure to increase the reimbursement for dialysis to meet the rising costs. The ESRD program has, in fact, been a model of economic efficiency with productivity increases offsetting the rising costs. When viewed from the outside, however, the economic benefits of delivering dialysis care seem to be ample, seen in the form of millionaire nephrologists and robust providers buying up facilities with the proceeds of productivity. A consequence of this improved productivity seen in shorter dialysis times and reuse of disposables appears to be an increase in mortality [6].

The human factor

Government restriction of reimbursement for dialysis is not the major problem contributing to preventable death in dialysis patients, however. The current reimbursement rate does not force the doctor to write a prescription for inadequate dialysis or to allow improper reuse. Moreover, failure of dialysis professionals to recognize deficiencies in the care of patients and develop as a result practice guidelines and standards, both individually and as a group, is not the fault of the government.

The problem of substandard care of dialysis patients frequently begins in the training of nephrologists. The art and science of dialysis is infrequently emphasized. Instead, many renal fellows are directed to 'important' clinical subspeciality areas such as transplantation, or biopsy diagnosis and immuno-suppressive treatment of renal disease, or laboratory endeavors involving animal kidneys. Taking care of hospitalized patients needing acute dialysis or having their blood access fixed is seen as neither exciting or important. They see dialysis prescribed by rote, with scant attention to individual patient needs. Serious attempts to assure the adequacy of treatment is rarely a priority. Habits and attitudes learned in training are often carried into practice. In addition, there is no reason to expect that those who spend several years of their training in the laboratory and a few months taking care of hospitalized dialysis patients are even remotely qualified to care for dialysis patients in an ambulatory setting. Yet this is where many find employment. The result: underdialysis by prescription, improper reprocessing of dialyzers, missed diagnoses and delayed correction of failing or malfunctioning blood access, overlooked signs or symptoms of malnutrition, failure to detect other treatable medical complications. These all contribute substantially to morbidity and mortality for hemodialysis patients. Yet this is the way things are and presumably the way they will continue.

Nephrologists do not shoulder the burden of responsibility alone. Many dialysis nurses today see themselves as automatons in a factory, putting patients on the machine and taking them off in a strictly regimented workaday schedule. This is in stark contrast to nurses of an earlier day who listened to patients and encouraged and taught them to do much for themselves. They were diagnosticians, reporting when patients were not well or accesses were not working properly, and often had the knowledge and latitude to do something about it. They provided the necessary safety net for diagnosis and prevention. True, doctors seemed more involved and appreciative of the nursing role in those days and they themselves were more interested in listening and learning and supporting a team effort. Perhaps this was because both doctors and nurses realized that they still had much to learn about this therapy. Today they think they know all they need to. As a result nurses come into dialysis today only for the job and if they stay it seems they do so for the security of a fixed and limited system of work and knowledge. Of those who remember the old days or have the interest and flexibility to know it can be better, a few struggle valiantly on, while others have escaped to jobs in industry or elsewhere.

Social workers have a place in this equation, more as victims than offenders. They are seen by many unit administrators as adjuncts of the billing department, whose only function is to ensure that the patients' medical coverage is up-to-date. This puts them inevitably at odds with the patient, when they should be working as patient advocate. They may not have time for their real work, burdened with the demands of administration and the assignment of too many patients. This is extremely unfortunate, because their work is vital to the adjustment of the renal patient to his new life. Compliance, survival and rehabilitation follow when the patients psychosocial needs are satisfied.

The often forgotten dietitian may be struggling to keep the patients on the restrictive predialysis diet, the only benefit to the patient being to minimize the symptoms of underdialysis. It certainly does not contribute to their good nutrition.

Add to today's dialysis facility mix the administrator, who makes the final decisions driven by the need of cost efficiency, which permits little time to meet human needs. Profit has become god in renal medicine. The irony is that poor care cuts into profit. When failure to prevent problems leads to hospitalization or premature death, the facility loses a valuable asset.

Nurses and patient care technicians can be trained in the detection of access problems and how to avoid infections. They can be involved in assuring the adequacy of dialysis treatments and achieving compliance to regimen by working with the patients.

It is true that many dialysis patients today are older and sicker and many are less appreciative of the privilege of having dialysis readily available as a life-saving treatment. This could account for part of the higher mortality rate, but also, and perhaps more so among these patients due to their lack of interest and participation in their treatment, preventable causes of death occur. The dictatorial conditions that exist in many dialysis units preclude patient involvement in their care.

Patients have been treated with maintenance hemodialysis for 33 years. There is a question that begs to be answered: Why then are there still no universally accepted standards of care?

Can the health and survival of hemodialysis patients be improved?

Emphatically yes, but the renal professional community, as a whole, needs to take the problem seriously. Doctors who are to care for dialysis patients must be trained and certified as skilled subspecialists in hemo and/or peritoneal dialysis as well as maintaining the skills of an internist. Nurses and patient care technicians must be given diagnostic training and take seriously the opportunity for application. Social workers must be freed to deal with the patients' psychosocial and economic problems as patient advocates. Dietitians must learn to preach adherence to a more liberal and practical dialysis diet supported by improved dialysis efficiency rather than promoting the excessively restricted predialysis diet. If they see it as being important to their survival, many patients can learn to take more control and thus assume greater responsibility for the outcome of their care. They must be allowed and encouraged to do so. If these steps are not pursued by professionals voluntarily to prevent avoidable dialysis morbidity and mortality, it should be assumed that patients will ask the Federal government to step in and require them to do so.

References

1. Held PJ, Brunner F, Odaka M, Garcia JR, Port FK, Gaylin DS. Five-year survival for end-stage renal disease patients in the United States, Europe, and Japan, 1982 to 1987. Am J Kidney Dis 1990; 15: 451–57.
2. Report on management of renal failure in Europe, XXII, 1991. Nephrol Dial Transplant 1992; 7: 16.
3. Plough AP, Salem S. Social and contextual factors in the analysis of mortality in end-stage renal disease patients: Implications for health policy. Am J Pub Health 1982; 72: 1293–95.
4. Lundin, AP. Recurrent uremic pericarditis: A mark of inadequate dialysis. Semin Dial 1990; 3: 5–6.
5. Held PJ, Blagg CR, Liska DW, Port FK, Hakim R, Levin N: The dose of hemodialysis according to dialysis prescription in Europe and the United States. Kidney Int 1992; 38: S16–21.
6. Held PJ, Levin NW, Bovbjerg RR, Pauly MV, Diamond LH. Mortality and duration of hemodialysis treatment. JAMA 1991; 265: 871–875.

CHAPTER 22

Lessons from mortality risks and rates

GEORGE E. SCHREINER

It seems agreed that annual mortality rates for dialysis patients reflect a considerable range from unit to unit, doctor to doctor, region to region and country to country. The US, starting late in its distribution efforts, without a system for universal health care, has done a remarkable feat in enabling close to 200,000 uremic patients to survive on dialysis at a unit cost which has steadily declined since 1973. Nothing else procured by our Government has declined in cost during those inflationary years. Moreover, the transplant rate has been the envy of many, limited mainly by the supply of organs and catering to many foreign-born nationals in the process.

None the less, the mortality countrywide in the US appears to be substantially higher than the rate predicted from good pilot studies. It is, regrettably, higher than that achieved in many other large and developed countries. It therefore behooves us to look critically into the program find what's wrong and then take the right steps to fix it. It is too simplistic to simply cite the case mix. The US program is too large to tolerate selection and so are many of its peer programs. By many probes, many correlations and many meetings, we have come to recognize some of the factors as shown in Table 1.

A recent statewide study of almost 4000 patients indicated that there may be a rank order of importance in the widely recognized risk factors. This order is shown in Table 2.

We need to ask: Why do non-dialyzed uremic patients die? The usual answer is that their clearances have slipped below critical levels. This often corresponds to a GFR range of 1 to 10, but there are many biologic

Table 1. General consensus on mortality risks

Age
Co-morbid conditions–ashd–cvd–pvd–dm–c–copd
Poor nutrition
HIV+<AIDS–13.2+/– 1.9 mos.
Non-AIDS–15.7 +/– 3 mos.
Depression–Psychological problems

205

E. A. Friedman (ed.), Death on Hemodialysis, 205–207.
© 1994 *Kluwer Academic Publishers.*

Table 2. Mortality rates rank order

1.	Older patients
2.	Whites
3.	Diabetic Nephropathy
4.	Angina
5.	Heart Failure
6.	Nutrition and function

N = 3612
Ann. Int. Med 1992; 117:332.

Table 3.

Kt/V	Patient wants early cut-off
Re-use	Staff wants early cut-off
Short dialysis	Financial incentives override

Why do dialyzed patients die? Perhaps their clearances have slowly slipped beneath a cumulative critical level. Since these levels are machine-sensitive and doctor-designed, why do we let them happen? Table 3 may provide some of the insights.

We need to ask: Has Kt/V become more of a cap than a safe minimum? Does re-use make dialysis less efficient? Has short dialysis become a euphemism for labor saving? Do staffs pander to the patient who has become impatient and irritable and fatigued? These may be the very symptoms of underdialysis. Do staff cut corners especially before weekends, holidays and mealtimes? Has the relentless ratcheting down of reimbursement made shortening of dialysis a quick route to profit or facility survival?

Perhaps it is time to get back to basics. The endocrinologists have it simple. Every patient is hyper.. hypo.. or 'eu'. Our basics are outlined in Table 4.

We know that large people with high lean body mass require a higher kidney function they need more dialysis. We know that people on high protein and in particular, binge diets need to raise their GFR and do! They need more dialysis. We know that people who are hyperthyroid, hyperthermic on heavy

Table 4. "EU PEE'

Body size & composition
Metabolism of diet
Metabolism of tissue
    Basal
    Fever
    Exercise
    Thyroid-growth hormone
Other causes of catabolism
    Time-Rhythm
    Clearance

exercise, have a high oxygen consumption or are growing, – require higher kidney function to stay "eu pee" – so do they need more dialysis. We know that catabolism is enhanced by infection, by disruptions of circadian rhythm and that high clearance machines may in themselves enhance catabolism. Wise dialyzers can learn basics from the kidneys God gave us!

Developments in Nephrology

1. J.S. Cheigh, K.H. Stenzel and A.L. Rubin (eds.): *Manual of Clinical Nephrology of the Rogosin Kidney Center.* 1981   ISBN 90-247-2397-3
2. K.D. Nolph (ed.): *Peritoneal Dialysis.* 1981 ed.: out of print
3rd revised and enlarged ed. 1988 (not in this series)   ISBN 0-89838-406-0
3. A.B. Gruskin and M.E. Norman (eds.): *Pediatric Nephrology.* 1981
     ISBN 90-247-2514-3
4. O. Schück: *Examination of the Kidney Function.* 1981   ISBN 0-89838-565-2
5. J. Strauss (ed.): *Hypertension, Fluid-electrolytes and Tubulopathies in Pediatric Nephrology.* 1982   ISBN 90-247-2633-6
6. J. Strauss (ed.): *Neonatal Kidney and Fluid-electrolytes.* 1983   ISBN 0-89838-575-X
7. J. Strauss (ed.): *Acute Renal Disorders and Renal Emergencies.* 1984
     ISBN 0-89838-663-2
8. L.J.A. Didio and P.M. Motta (eds.): *Basic, Clinical, and Surgical Nephrology.* 1985
     ISBN 0-89838-698-5
9. E.A. Friedman and C.M. Peterson (eds.): *Diabetic Nephropathy.* Strategy for Therapy. 1985   ISBN 0-89838-735-3
10. R. Dzúrik, B. Lichardus and W. Guder: *Kidney Metabolism and Function.* 1985
     ISBN 0-89838-749-3
11. J. Strauss (ed.): *Homeostasis, Nephrotoxicy, and Renal Anomalies in the Newborn.* 1986   ISBN 0-89838-766-3
12. D.G. Oreopoulos (ed.): *Geriatric Nephrology.* 1986   ISBN 0-89838-781-7
13. E.P. Paganini (ed.): *Acute Continuous Renal Replacement Therapy.* 1986
     ISBN 0-89838-793-0
14. J.S. Cheigh, K.H. Stenzel and A.L. Rubin (eds.): *Hypertension in Kidney Disease.* 1986
     ISBN 0-89838-797-3
15. N. Deane, R.J. Wineman and G.A. Benis (eds.): *Guide to Reprocessing of Hemodialyzers.* 1986   ISBN 0-89838-798-1
16. C. Ponticelli, L. Minetti and G. D'Amico (eds.): *Antiglobulins, Cryoglobulins and Glomerulonephritis.* 1986   ISBN 0-89838-810-4
17. J. Strauss (ed.) with the assistence of L. Strauss: *Persistent Renalgenitourinary Disorders.* 1987   ISBN 0-89838-845-7
18. V.E. Andreucci and A. Dal Canton (eds.): *Diuretics.* Basic, Pharmacological, and Clinical Aspects. 1987   ISBN 0-89838-885-6
19. P.H. Bach and E.H. Lock (eds.): *Nephrotoxicity in the Experimental and Clinical Situation,* Part 1. 1987   ISBN 0-89838-997-1
20. P.H. Bach and E.H. Lock (eds.): *Nephrotoxicity in the Experimental and Clinical Situation,* Part 2. 1987   ISBN 0-89838-980-2
21. S.M. Gore and B.A. Bradley (eds.): *Renal Transplantation.* Sense and Sensitization. 1988   ISBN 0-89838-370-6
22. L. Minetti, G. D'Amico and C. Ponticelli: *The Kidney in Plasma Cell Dyscrasias.* 1988
     ISBN 0-89838-385-4
23. A.S. Lindblad, J.W. Novak and K.D. Nolph (eds.): *Continuous Ambulatory Peritoneal Dialysis in the USA.* Final Report of the National CAPD Registry 1981–1988. 1989
     ISBN 0-7923-0179-X

Developments in Nephrology

Kluwer Academic Publishers – Dordrecht / Boston / London

The manufacturer's authorised representative in the EU is Springer
Nature Customer Service Centre GmbH, Europaplatz 3, 69115 Heidelberg,
Germany. If you have any concerns regarding our products, please
contact ProductSafety@springernature.com

Printed and bound by CPI Group (UK) Ltd, Croydon, CR0 4YY
24/04/2026
02096348-0003